MW01252836

Translating Expertise

MEDICAL LIBRARY ASSOCIATION BOOKS

The Medical Library Association (MLA) features books that showcase the expertise of health sciences librarians for other librarians and professionals.

MLA Books are excellent resources for librarians in hospitals, medical research practice, and other settings. These volumes will provide health-care professionals and patients with accurate information that can improve outcomes and save lives.

Each book in the series has been overseen editorially since conception by the Medical Library Association Books Panel, composed of MLA members with expertise spanning the breadth of health sciences librarianship.

Medical Library Association Books Panel

Lauren M. Young, AHIP, chair
Kristen L. Young, AHIP, chair designate
Michel C. Atlas
Dorothy C. Ogdon, AHIP
Karen McElfresh, AHIP
Megan Curran Rosenbloom
Tracy Shields, AHIP
JoLinda L. Thompson, AHIP
Heidi Heilemann, AHIP, board liaison

About the Medical Library Association

Founded in 1898, MLA is a 501(c)(3) nonprofit, educational organization of 3,500 individual and institutional members in the health sciences information field that provides lifelong educational opportunities, supports a knowledge base of health information research, and works with a global network of partners to promote the importance of quality information for improved health to the health-care community and the public.

Books in Series

The Medical Library Association Guide to Providing Consumer and Patient Health Information edited by Michele Spatz
Health Sciences Librarianship edited by M. Sandra Wood
Curriculum-Based Library Instruction: From Cultivating Faculty Relationships Assessment edited by Amy Blevins and Megan Inman
Mobile Technologies for Every Library by Ann Whitney Gleason
Marketing for Special and Academic Libraries: A Planning and Best Practices Sourcebook by Patricia Higginbottom and Valerie Gordon
Translating Expertise: The Librarian's Role in Translational Research edited by Marisa L. Conte

Translating Expertise

The Librarian's Role in Translational Research

Edited by Marisa L. Conte

ROWMAN & LITTLEFIELD
Lanham • Boulder • New York • London

Published by Rowman & Littlefield
A wholly owned subsidiary of The Rowman & Littlefield Publishing Group, Inc.
4501 Forbes Boulevard, Suite 200, Lanham, Maryland 20706
www.rowman.com

Unit A, Whitacre Mews, 26-34 Stannary Street, London SE11 4AB

British Library Cataloguing in Publication Information Available

Library of Congress Cataloging-in-Publication Data

Name: Conte, Marisa L., 1976–, editor.
Title: Translating expertise : the librarian's role in translational research / edited by Marisa L.
  Conte.
Other titles: Medical Library Association books.
Description: Lanham : Rowman & Littlefield, [2016] | Series: Medical Library Association
  books | Includes bibliographical references and index.
Identifiers: LCCN 2016010729| ISBN 9781442262676 (hardcover : alk. paper) | ISBN
  9781442262683 (electronic)
Subjects: | MESH: Clinical and Translational Science Awards (Program). | Translational
  Medical Research | Librarians | Professional Role
Classification: LCC R119.5 | NLM W 20.55.T7 | DDC 026/.61—dc23 LC record
  available at https://lccn.loc.gov/2016010729

Printed in the United States of America

I dedicate this work with respect and gratitude to Lothar Spang, Barbara Rapp, and Jane Blumenthal, whose mentorship made it possible, and to Tim Neville and Jean Song, whose support made it happen. Also, with much love, to my parents, Gail and Mike, who always expected to see my name on the cover of a book.

Contents

Preface

Health sciences libraries have undergone numerous changes in recent years. Many of these stories are already familiar to the reader: resources have shifted from paper to electronic; increased costs paired with budget constraints have affected our abilities to provide access to these resources; the physical footprint of many libraries is being reduced or eliminated to satisfy other institutional needs; and both libraries and librarians are looking for new ways to demonstrate relevance and leverage valuable knowledge and skills. In addition to dealing with a dynamic information environment, health sciences libraries are also responding to changes in the biomedical education and research environments.

This book tells the story of how librarians have engaged with the biomedical research community as it shifted to embrace translational science via the Clinical and Translational Science Award (CTSA) program, funded by the National Institutes of Health (NIH) since 2006. The CTSA program, which currently provides funding to more than sixty institutions, was intended to reengineer the clinical research enterprise at the institutional level, speeding the time from preclinical discovery to the development of therapies to improve human health. The CTSA program has emphasized team science and the development of infrastructures to share information and resources among research partners across the country, facilitating new collaborations and increasing research capacity in both preclinical and clinical contexts.

Although the CTSA has been the model for basic and clinical research for almost a decade, it can still be difficult to understand the scope and breadth of translational research. This book begins by providing a historical background of and context for the CTSA program, including the impact of recent administrative changes. As universities have competed for CTSA funding and often developed or recalibrated institutional infrastructures and research support services to support successful awards, the face of biomedical research has changed. These changes (and their intended and unintended consequences) introduced new roles for health sciences librarians, creating novel opportunities to engage with researchers, research administrators, and community members as active partners in the research enterprise.

Examples of the paths librarians took to identify these opportunities and create or fill these new roles are the highlight of this book. The goals are to identify entry points to engaging with the translational research enterprise at various levels and to describe the development of services and resources to address the needs of everyone involved with translational science: researchers, administrators, and the public. Presented as case studies, these examples show how librarians identify institutional needs and develop relevant programs and relationships in areas from collection development, instruction, and compliance to assessment. They also showcase librarians' creativity in developing and maintaining relationships with researchers. These case studies are examples of not only best practices in the integration of traditional librarian skill sets into the research enterprise but also lessons learned as librarians identified newly emerging opportunities to leverage skills in information organization and dissemination in the context of translational research.

No book about librarians can ever claim (or hope!) to be comprehensive; the field of health sciences librarianship is full of creative and talented people who continually seek new ways to spread knowledge and build connections by applying their skills in information management, organization, and retrieval. It is my hope that, in presenting examples of the work of librarians from multiple institutions who have integrated in translational science in a variety of ways, this book will inspire librarians looking for ways to engage the translational research audiences at their institutions, as well as those who are already participating in translational research (with or without a designated CTSA program).

1

Libraries Supporting the Translational Science Spectrum

An Introduction

Kristi L. Holmes

BACKGROUND AND PERSPECTIVE

In 2006, the National Institutes of Health (NIH) launched the Clinical and Translational Science Award (CTSA) program. The goal of the CTSA program is to create an academic home and provide valuable support for infrastructure and collaboration to facilitate clinical and translational research initiatives across the United States.[1] Originally administered through the National Center for Research Resources (NCRR), the CTSA program is now housed in the National Center for Advancing Translational Sciences (NCATS).[2]

The CTSA program provides funding for the establishment and support of more than sixty competitively awarded centers dedicated to translational research.[3] The hubs themselves are transinstitutional collaborations and often feature partnerships with other institutions, community organizations, and industry. This network of biomedical research institutes works both independently and in concert to advance the CTSA's programmatic goals:

- Train and cultivate the translational science workforce;
- Engage patients and communities in every phase of the translational process;
- Promote the integration of special and underserved populations in translational research across the human life span;
- Innovate processes to increase the quality and efficiency of translational research, particularly of multisite trials; and
- Advance the use of cutting-edge informatics.

Additionally, special emphasis has been placed on the concept of "team science" since the CTSA program's inception with the objective of implementing more efficient and effective processes to accomplish program goals. Multidisciplinary, collaborative teams composed of members with diverse roles and perspectives are a hallmark of a healthy clinical and translational science (CTS) enterprise.

WHAT IS TRANSLATIONAL SCIENCE?

The CTSA program is, by nature, a very large and cross-cutting effort to translate research discoveries more efficiently and effectively, ultimately resulting in improved health of our communities. The National Center for Advancing Translational Sciences defines translation as "the process of turning observations in the laboratory, clinic and community into interventions that improve the health of individuals and the public—from diagnostics and therapeutics to medical procedures and behavioral changes" and the concept of translational science as "the field of investigation focused on understanding the scientific and operational principles underlying each step of the translational process."[4]

Clinical and translational sciences (CTSs) are often represented linearly (figure 1.1) and described in terms such as "from the bench to the bedside and beyond." The reality of CTS necessitates more than a unidirectional arrow, however; both forward and reverse interactions along the "spectrum"[5] are critical for success. For example, research discoveries spur medical device development and application of therapies—feedback from which informs further basic science research and development—and can also be applied to better enable successful clinical trials.

This concept of translating discoveries is relevant across all aspects of biomedicine and beyond. As such, translational research is not limited to CTSA-funded programs; it is also happening across the different institutes at NIH in the form of both extramurally supported projects and on-site intermural research. Translational research is also accomplished at research institutes, within stand-alone hospitals, and at schools of veterinary medicine, engineering, communication, and business. Translational research can only realize its full potential by engaging and encouraging

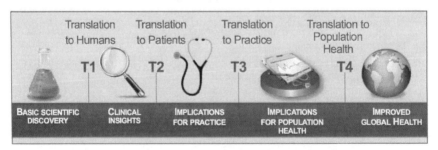

Figure 1.1. Adapted from the Medical University of South Carolina's News from Nexus, http://academicdepartments.musc.edu/sctr/nexus/news.

diverse voices and perspectives. Indeed, community-engaged research is making important strides as research is translated (or disseminated) away from the academic research environment and into our community clinics, community centers, retirement facilities, and schools. This is an exciting area of work, and improvements in process, engagement, and dissemination should lead to real improvements in public health.

CHANGES IN THE CTSA PROGRAM

The National Institutes of Health, at the recommendation of Congress, requested a study by the Institute of Medicine (IOM) in 2012. The IOM (renamed the National Academy of Medicine in 2015)[6] convened a committee to review the mission and strategic goals of the CTSA program. The committee's report, delivered in 2013, established targeted recommendations to guide the program and also described key opportunities for action to ensure future success (textbox 1.1). Key findings of the report include recognition that the CTSA program makes significant contributions toward the advancement of clinical and translational research and several recommendations for revisions to the program to make it more efficient and effective. These revisions were intended to help ensure future successes and clearly establish the CTSA program as the national leader for advancing CTS.[7]

TEXTBOX 1.1
Institute of Medicine Recommendations

Recommendations by the IOM committee for next steps for the CTSA program and opportunities for advancing clinical and translational research include the following:

- Strengthen NCATS leadership of the CTSA program
- Reconfigure and streamline the CTSA consortium
- Build on the strengths of individual CTSAs across the spectrum of clinical and translational research
- Formalize and standardize evaluation processes for individual CTSAs and the CTSA program
- Advance innovation in education and training programs
- Ensure community engagement in all phases of research
- Strengthen clinical and translational research relevant to child health

---

NIH gathered an expert team to address the findings in the IOM report. In a statement in response to the IOM report, *The CTSA Program at NIH: Opportunities for Advancing Clinical and Translational Research*, NCATS director Christopher P. Austin, MD, described the next steps:

First, NCATS will increase its direct and active leadership of the program while assembling a working group of NCATS Advisory Council members and other key

stakeholders to advise me on implementation of the report's recommendations. Designation of clear, measurable goals and objectives that address critical issues across the
full spectrum of clinical and translational research will be one of our first tasks.

Second, the committee's recommendation to reconfigure and streamline CTSA program governance will result in a more efficiently managed program. This process also
will begin immediately and in coordination with stakeholders.[8]

NCATS immediately established the Advisory Council Working Group (ACWG) on
the IOM Report: The CTSA Program at NIH[9] to provide support on incorporating
these recommendations. The ACWG also established a set of goals for the CTSA
program that both reflect the recommendations of the IOM report and establish
meaningful changes to help power CTS forward:

- Workforce development. The translational science workforce has the skills and
  knowledge necessary to advance translation of discoveries.
- Collaboration/engagement. Stakeholders are engaged in collaborations to advance translation.
- Integration. Translational science is integrated across its multiple phases and
  disciplines within complex populations and across the individual life span.
- Methods/processes. The scientific study of the process of conducting translational science itself enables significant advances in translation.

Processes across the CTSA consortium and mechanisms for engagement by the different hubs were also restructured to provide a more streamlined workflow, enhance
the efficiencies of the program, and foster collaboration. Originally, five strategic
goal committees and a series of fourteen working groups, called the key function
committees, provided the organizational process structure of the CTSAs. The CTSA
program restructuring created a more streamlined structure directly linked to the
ACWG's goals, now advanced in large part by five new domain task forces (DTFs).
The DTFs are based on the four strategic goals established by the ACWG: workforce
development, collaboration/engagement, integration, and methods/processes, plus
the key infrastructure emphasis area of informatics.[10] Each NCATS-funded hub has
one seat on each DTF. The DTFs are also fairly streamlined; each group is led by
a five-person leadership team, and each DTF facilitates ad hoc work through up to
five work groups (figure 1.2).[11]

TRANSLATING THE RECOMMENDATIONS FOR THE FUTURE

The IOM recommendations are pushing NCATS toward a successful future for
CTS. They have shaped both the governance and the functional structure of the
CTSA consortium and even influenced the funding announcement from NCATS.
The best example of this can be seen in the first request for applications (RFAs)
from NCATS after the incorporation of the recommendations, which was released

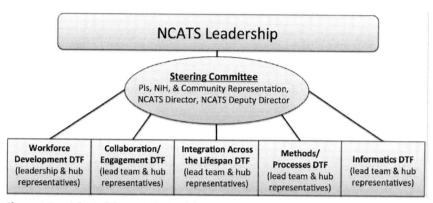

Figure 1.2. Adapted from NCATS Advisory Council Working Group.

on September 12, 2014.[12] The new RFA strongly reflects the recent work within NCATS, by both providing some background and context and supporting the recommendations outlined in the IOM report and the input from the ACWG.[11] As stated in the RFA, "With the goal of catalyzing the development of methods and technologies that lead to more efficient translation of biomedical discoveries into interventions shown to improve health, NCATS is evolving the CTSA program into an integrated research and training environment for clinical and translational sciences that aims to dramatically improve efficiency and quality across the translational research spectrum."[12] The new RFA has a different structure than seen previously, with reorganized sections combined with new components to better delineate the required components of the application necessary to meet this vision. This RFA was reissued on July 23, 2015.[13]

LIBRARY VOICES

Meeting the goals of CTS is a huge challenge. As shown above, and as libraries know all too well, the modern academic medical environment is becoming increasingly complex to navigate in terms of both organizational structure and process. Additionally, the sheer quantity of information and data generated on a daily basis as a result of biomedical research is astounding. This flood of data is a double-edged sword, generating great opportunities for discovery, but making meaningful discovery a challenging process.

Libraries and librarians are uniquely positioned to help address some of these challenges. We are fortunate to have as role models many insightful and creative libraries working in support of CTS, several of which are included in this book. In the following chapters you will find dynamic examples of engagement across the translational spectrum, indeed "from the bench to the bedside and beyond." These programs, services, and partnerships are examples of what can happen when core library strengths intersect with key needs in the operational workflow of translational sciences institutes.

The chapters that follow have been organized to represent work in the basic sciences, open science, community engagement, education support, networking and collaboration, and infrastructure. These library-based programs are good models to emulate and can inspire thoughtful development of programs from many different types of medical libraries. In this book you will find the following:

- Basic sciences such as bioinformatics;
- Open-source tools to facilitate clinical research, including tranSMART, a translational data-sharing and analysis platform, and REDCap, secure software for data capture and management;
- Community engagement and service including support for a community research fellowship training program and partnerships with the public library to integrate information services and support deep within the community;
- Education support and services placed within the clinical and translational sciences institute;
- Facilitated connections in big and small ways through libraries' work with research networking tools and through innovative programs;
- Infrastructure, including projects to help make resources and services more discoverable, the changing role of the library in support of the translational research enterprise, and leveraging key library resources to support objectives of the Clinical and Translational Sciences Institute; and
- Innovative library-based programs and services that not only support but also accelerate local and national evaluation and assessment activities.

WHY LIBRARIES? AND WHY LIBRARIANS?

Libraries are perfectly poised to support and partner with CTS in the form of both traditional library resources and services and specialty information services. More and more, this specialty information support work is conducted by a growing cadre of diverse information specialists often called "informationists." Librarians have served key roles across academic medical campuses and on clinical teams for a long time. The informationist takes this concept one step forward, placing the information professional in a position to work in direct partnership with CTS teams. The informationist concept can be more than a description of the work that libraries already do; it can also be a tool to help convey possible opportunities for partnerships and library integration in a manner that can be easier for the CTS team to envision. The work of Davidoff and Florance[14] as well as a commentary by Plutchak[15] provided valuable perspective to me when I joined the medical library and enabled me to envision my role as a real partner on projects and initiatives. While these two papers were published more than fifteen years ago, I believe they still provide critical context and encouragement for librarians who are shaping new roles in specialty information support.

Many of the programs and partnerships described within these pages reflect specialty services and expertise by the library team as they integrate with CTS workflows. A number of libraries have successfully expanded the informationist concept in bright, bold new ways, most notably the NIH Library,[16] Welch Medical Library at Johns Hopkins University,[17] the Eskind Biomedical Library at Vanderbilt University,[18] and the Taubman Health Sciences Library at the University of Michigan.[19] These successful programs are mature and involve several informationists; however, important programs and services often begin with a single idea or person.[20,21,22]

Attention is often paid to the credentials of information scientists that are based in libraries. To be sure, librarians and library staff with advanced science degrees are able to offer a different level of support to the basic science community than someone who may not have a research or basic science background. However, libraries without this internal expertise can still play a critical role in supporting CTS on campus. Education and training can be a good place to start; education and workforce development is a priority area for CTS institutes, and libraries are often already engaged in educational support activities, making it easier to realize some early successes. Examples of library activities in support of education and workforce development include developing and supporting a lecture series with campus partners, hosting vendor workshops for researchers, and participating in research events on campus to share information about library services.

Finally, libraries can be great partners to help catalyze campus initiatives.[23] The library is a trusted and impartial organization on campus with a long tradition of service and support of all missions of the institution. This perspective provides a great opportunity for libraries to bring their resources and expertise to CTS teams. Libraries often have information-technology (IT) and data expertise among the librarians and library staff, opening new opportunities for services and partnerships. Additionally, librarians have many other skills, abilities, and talents that can support various aspects of CTS activities, including domain knowledge or subject expertise, information structure and organization, instructional design, and an understanding of the local research, clinical, and education landscapes. Their close and trusted relationships with clients enable librarians to understand and meet the needs of their users. Librarians also know how to bring people together and are often called upon to be a matchmaker for clients as well as to play a role on various collaboration and networking information-technology projects on campus.

GETTING STARTED

Getting involved with a translational research enterprise can seem intimidating, not least because there are so many different aspects to consider: the many people and groups within the organization and beyond, as well as priorities and key areas of emphasis for the individual organization, the CTSA consortium, and the larger bio-medical research community. Given the complex nature of both CTS and the local and national infrastructures, it can be difficult to understand how our libraries can get involved, what expertise we can bring to the table, and how we can communicate this expertise and introduce ourselves, and our resources and services, in a manner that guarantees the library a seat at the table moving forward.

Libraries may choose to meet this challenge in a variety of ways—from reconfig-uring existing staff and resources incrementally to hiring new, specialized informa-tionist positions and making major investments in research software or computing infrastructure to support the research enterprise. In addition to resource allocation, there are several things that libraries can do to grow partnership opportunities, expand our programming and services, and support local translational science initiatives in a manner that reflects institutional priorities both within CTS and beyond. Perhaps most importantly, consider your local environment in terms of both priorities of the transitional sciences institute and existing skills and resources within your library. Look for opportunities that both play to these strengths and enhance the library's ability to support the campus, rather than creating services that will only benefit a small area of CTS research at the expense of a large com-mitment of librarians' time and efforts.

IDENTIFYING STAKEHOLDERS

Stakeholders are a critical piece of the puzzle. It is important to understand who is leading CTS initiatives and also who may be able to open doors for the library. If your institution already has a CTS institute, a visit to that institute's website (linked to on the CTSA program hub site) is a good first step. Study the leadership roster and the roles and responsibilities of individuals involved to become better informed of the structure of your local CTS organization and to gain a perspective of possible areas of collaboration. Check to see if there are people who are ongoing friends and supporters of the library, as they can often be a good way to become involved. What if there is no translational science institute at your university or in your organiza-tion? That doesn't mean that translational research isn't happening! Reach out to colleagues who might be able to help you identify key areas of library involvement. Search the literature for publications about translational projects from your institu-tion and reach out to these investigators.

LEARN ABOUT PRIORITIES AND PAIN POINTS

Becoming familiar with key local and national initiatives will allow you to develop and align services and resources to more effectively meet potential need areas. A number of "Issues in Translation" have been identified that NCATS aims to address:

- Predictive efficacy and toxicology;
- De-risking therapeutic development;
- Clinical research efficiency;
- Collaboration and partnerships; and
- Data transparency and release.[24]

Libraries should think about these and other possible "pain points"—many of these actually match well with library expertise, such as publication tracking and evaluation, compliance issues, dissemination, and support for education and training. Brainstorm about these pain points as an entrée to conversations for future projects and also do an honest and positive assessment of the types of amazing expertise that libraries can bring to the table.

In addition to leveraging existing strengths, librarians should be encouraged to learn about the many moving parts of modern translational medicine. A straightforward manner of accomplishing this includes subscribing to tables of contents from relevant journals and finding new ways to stay current with journal content. Journals provide high-level discussions of content in the commentary, perspectives, and notes sections that often address CTS topics. Some of the best sources for this perspective can be found in journals such as *Science, Science Translational Medicine, Clinical and Translational Medicine, Nature,* and the suite of journals at the Public Library of Science (PLoS). Librarians can also subscribe to newsfeeds of NIH news releases or blogs of authors who are working in support of or who are interested in translational medicine. The NCATS home page[25] and the CTSA program home page[26] are wonderful resources for background and perspective on the topic of translational science and help establish a vision for the future. The CTSA consortium site[27] is also a great source of information and serves as the go-to place for announcements, notes, and slides from meetings, and even timely updates on critical topics with support materials, such as the CTSA Common Metrics Booklet.[28] Finally, libraries should look locally to learn about translational medicine too. Identify campus-wide initiatives related to clinical and translational science and reach out to participants and stakeholders.

A good way to get to know people on campus is by engaging them in their environments and building upon activities that often happen in the context of liaison work. Examples include attending research seminars, grand rounds, workshops, and campus events where librarians can learn about ongoing research on campus and even view posters and have conversations with the scientists as they present their work. These conversations may seem less intimidating when you realize that researchers won't expect you to be an expert in every detail of their science. A meaningful conversation with the researcher can include a chat about what it is like for them as they try to accomplish work on campus. What are their greatest individual pain points? What opportunities are there for the library to get more involved in their work, whether it's the work of their center or their department? Are there ways that the library can better support their students or other trainees?

TEXTBOX 1.2
Eight Tips for Getting Started with CTS

1. Do your homework. Identify stakeholders, audience, and local champions.
2. Develop ways of monitoring local and national/global issues.
3. Brainstorm and complete a gap analysis. What's missing? What role can the library play? Are you already doing work that might be described as supporting CTS?
4. Develop your own timeline. What can you do today? Next week? In a year? Long term?
5. Employ strategic planning. What resources and expertise do you have in hand? What do you need?
6. Communicate. Develop a clear message to communicate with your campus and CTS stakeholders to encourage engagement and partnerships.
7. Don't wait to move forward on CTS efforts. Waiting until you have a new hire or more resources may delay your work indefinitely. Small successes can lead to additional resources and opportunities for the library.
8. Be generous and persistent. Communicate opportunities for collaboration to CTS stakeholders. Look for ways to address critical needs (such as support for compliance) and be kindly persistent. Keep communicating, as stakeholders are faced with many competing priorities that may make it difficult to hear the library message sometimes.

KINDRED SPIRITS AND OPPORTUNITIES FOR THE FUTURE

Clinical and translational sciences institutes and libraries are ideal partners. We've had an opportunity to see this in action at Northwestern University, where the value of this natural partnership has been amplified in some interesting ways. In 2013, Galter Health Sciences Library was administratively moved into the reporting structure of the Northwestern University Clinical and Translational Sciences (NUCATS) Institute. Galter Library received immediate and real benefits from this arrangement, including research administration support and opportunities for engagement through work groups and project partnerships. We also benefit from a team of advocates at NUCATS who promote the library and library services with unending enthusiasm through NUCATS newsletters, weekly messages to campus, social media messages, and in presentations across campus and for partner organizations.

Libraries and CTS institutes are truly kindred spirits; both function as components of core infrastructure, partnering with others to facilitate successful progress toward the research, clinical care, community engagement, and educational missions of the organization. We enthusiastically anticipate more opportunities for continued growth as a result of our ongoing work with NUCATS and believe that this also holds true for other medical libraries as they partner with their local CTS community. Libraries and our expertise are more important than ever, and the examples of library programs and partnerships contained in this book underscore this important contribution.

NOTES

1. National Center for Advancing Translational Sciences. About the CTSA program. 2015. http://www.ncats.nih.gov/ctsa/about. Accessed January 8, 2016.

2. Rockey S. Working through the transitions of NCRR and NCATS. 2012. https://nexus.od.nih.gov/all/2012/01/06/working-through-the-transitions-of-ncrr-and-ncats. Accessed January 8, 2016.

3. National Center for Advancing Translational Sciences. CTSA program hubs. 2015. http://www.ncats.nih.gov/ctsa/about/hubs. Accessed January 8, 2016.

4. National Center for Advancing Translational Sciences. About translation. 2015. http://www.ncats.nih.gov/translation. Accessed January 8, 2016.

5. National Center for Advancing Translational Sciences. Translational science spectrum. 2015. https://ncats.nih.gov/translation/spectrum. Accessed January 21, 2016.

6. National Academy of Sciences. Press release: Institute of Medicine to become National Academy of Medicine. 2015. http://iom.nationalacademies.org/Global/News%20Announcements/IOM-to-become-NAM-Press-Release.aspx#sthash.mOvqLvRX.dpuf. Accessed January 8, 2016.

7. Institute of Medicine. *The CTSA Program at NIH: Opportunities for Advancing Clinical and Translational Research.* Washington, DC: National Academies Press; 2013.

8. National Center for Advancing Translational Sciences. NCATS director statement: Institute of Medicine report on the CTSA program at NIH. 2013. http://ncats.nih.gov/news/releases/2013/ctsa-iom-statement. Accessed January 8, 2016.

9. National Center for Advancing Translational Sciences. Council working group on the IOM report: The CTSA program at NIH. 2015. https://ncats.nih.gov/advisory/council/subcomm/ctsaiom. Accessed January 8, 2016.

10. National Center for Advancing Translational Sciences. Domain task forces. 2015. https://ctsacentral.org/consortium/domain-task-forces. Accessed January 8, 2016.

11. National Center for Advancing Translational Sciences NCATS advisory council working group on the IOM report: The CTSA program at NIH, a working group of the NCATS advisory council to the director. Bethesda, MD: NCATS; 2014.

12. National Institutes of Health. RFA-TR-14-009. 2014. http://grants.nih.gov/grants/guide/rfa-files/RFA-TR-14-009.html. Accessed January 8, 2016.

13. National Institutes of Health. PA-15-304. 2015. http://grants.nih.gov/grants/guide/pa-files/PAR-15-304.html. Accessed January 8, 2016.

14. Davidoff F, Florance V. The informationist: A new health profession? *Ann Intern Med.* 2000 Jun 20;132(12):996–98.

15. Plutchak TS. Informationists and librarians. *Bull Med Libr Assoc.* 2000;88(4):391–92.

16. National Institutes of Health Library. Informationists. 2015. http://nihlibrary.nih.gov/Services/Pages/Informationists.aspx. Accessed January 8, 2016.

17. William H. Welch Medical Library, Johns Hopkins University School of Medicine. The Welch Library embedded informationist program. 2015. http://welch.jhmi.edu/welchone/The-Welch-Library-Embedded-Informationist-Program. Accessed January 8, 2016.

18. Annette and Irwin Eskind Biomedical Library, Vanderbilt University Medical Center. Knowledge management. 2015. http://www.mc.vanderbilt.edu/km. Accessed January 8, 2016.

19. A. Alfred Taubman Health Sciences Library. University of Michigan. Informationists. 2015. http://www.lib.umich.edu/taubman-health-sciences-library/informationists. Accessed January 8, 2016.

20. Henderson ME, Knott, TL. Starting a research data management program based in a university library. *Med Ref Serv Q.* 2015;34(1):47–59.

21. Federer L. The librarian as research informationist: A case study. *J Med Libr Assoc.* 2013;101(4):298–302.

22. Holmes KL, Lyon JA, Johnson LM, Sarli CC, Tennant MR. Library-based clinical and translational research support. *J Med Libr Assoc.* 2013;101(4):326–35.

23. Garcia-Milian R, Norton HF, Auten B, Davis VI, Holmes KL, Johnson M, Tennant MR. Librarians as part of cross-disciplinary, multi-institutional team projects: Experiences from the VIVO collaboration. *Sci Technol Libr.* 2013;32(2):160–75.

24. National Center for Advancing Translational Sciences. Issues in translation. 2015. https://ncats.nih.gov/translation/issues. Accessed January 8, 2016.

25. National Center for Advancing Translational Sciences. Home page. 2016. http://www .ncats.nih.gov/. Accessed January 8, 2016.

26. National Center for Advancing Translational Sciences. The Clinical and Translational Science Award (CTSA) program. 2016. https://ncats.nih.gov/ctsa. Accessed January 8, 2016.

27. Clinical and Translational Science Awards (CTSA) Consortium. CTSA Central. 2016. https://ctsacentral.org/. Accessed January 8, 2016.

28. National Center for Advancing Translational Sciences. CTSA program common metrics. 2015. https://ctsacentral.org/wp-content/uploads/CTSA-Common-Metrics-Book let-12-16-2015.pdf. Accessed January 8, 2016.

2

Bioinformatics Projects with the Clinical and Translational Sciences Institute

Building Success Step by Step

Pamela L. Shaw

INTRODUCTION

Northwestern University

Northwestern University is a private institution established in 1850 to serve the Northwest Territory of the United States. It was founded on the shores of Lake Michigan in an area that later became the town of Evanston, Illinois. The university now includes three campuses: the main campus in Evanston, Illinois; the Chicago campus, home to the medical and law schools; and a campus in Doha, Qatar.[1]

The Feinberg School of Medicine and Galter Health Sciences Library

Northwestern's medical school began in 1859 as the medical department of Lind University. The medical school grew through numerous changes and expansions and became known as the Feinberg School of Medicine in 2002.[2] The medical library grew with each expansion of the medical school until a gift from Jack and Dollie Galter led to renovation and expansion in 1994–1996 and the designation of the library as Galter Health Sciences Library.[3]

NUCATS: Northwestern University Clinical and Translational Sciences Institute

The Northwestern University Clinical and Translational Sciences (NUCATS) Institute was founded in 2007 and received a thirty-million-dollar Clinical and Translational Science Award (CTSA) from the National Institutes of Health (NIH) in 2008. It serves as a source for Clinical and Translational Science (CTS) support and funding for Northwestern University and its clinical partners, supporting seven schools at Northwestern and three clinical affiliates.[4]

In 2013, the Galter Health Sciences Library underwent an administrative infrastructure change and came under the management of NUCATS. Many events led to this change, beginning with the hiring of a new dean of the Feinberg School of Medicine in 2011. The dean had a strong set of goals for the school to expand the clinical and translational research enterprise. In keeping with these goals, the dean believed that Galter Library should expand its involvement in bio- and medical informatics support and training. The most logical administrative governance division for the library would be under the leadership of NUCATS, specifically, working in close partnership with the deputy director of NUCATS, who is also the chair of the Division of Health and Biomedical Informatics for the Department of Preventive Medicine at Feinberg. This change made Galter Library the first medical library to be a division of a university's clinical and translational science institute. Though Galter is a division of NUCATS, the library supports the entire medical school community, and we maintain a budget and staff that are managed by the library, with our own director and administration.

NUCATS has a history of robust clinical and bioinformatics programs; these have undergone numerous changes through the years. Northwestern's Chicago-based bioinformatics initiatives worked under the moniker Bioinformatics Consulting Core, supported by the Robert H. Lurie Comprehensive Cancer Center and Northwestern's Biomedical Informatics Center (NUBIC), a core of NUCATS. Later, the bioinformatics components were separated from medical informatics into the Bioinformatics Research Collaboratory (BIRC) of NUCATS. BIRC was then integrated into NUCATS's Quantitative Methods Group, and its services and functions were renamed the Advanced Bioinformatics and Bio-Computing (ABBC) Core under new leadership in 2014. NUCATS informatics administrators still tend to refer to informatics units under the NUBIC name, but molecular and clinical functions and cores are managed by distinct entities.

BIOINFORMATICS IN LIBRARIES AND CTSAS, AND BIOINFORMATICS AT NUCATS

Library-based bioinformatics experts are becoming more common; many libraries now employ librarians with advanced basic science degrees or nonlibrarian informatics experts who support bioinformatics and basic sciences from the library.[5-16] My position at Galter Library was created in 2005, based on the model described by Michele Tennant,[7] when Galter was looking to expand its basic science support and to establish bioinformatics support from the library.

At the time I completed my master of science in library and information science (MSLIS) in December 2005, I had been working as a laboratory technician at

Northwestern's Feinberg School of Medicine since 1993. My involvement with the Northwestern research community was attractive to Galter administration, since I had both a personal history and overall familiarity with research infrastructure at the medical school. I was hired as biosciences librarian at Galter beginning in January 2006. However, I did not have a degree in bioinformatics, and my bachelor's degree in neuroscience was almost twenty years old.

When I applied for the position at Galter, I demonstrated the use of the National Center for Biotechnology Information's (NCBI) basic local alignment search tool (BLAST) during the interview process, but my overall knowledge of bioinformatics was limited. My experience as a laboratory technician was largely in anatomy, pathology, and immunohistochemistry, with very little molecular technique required. One of the roles for the biosciences librarian position was to support researchers in the use of bioinformatics tools and databases, so Galter's associate director encouraged me to pursue a second graduate degree in computational biology or bioinformatics. I was open to the idea because bioinformatics and biostatistics were areas of research that were fascinating to me. Northwestern University offered a master's program in computational biology and bioinformatics (CBB) that had a small graduate student cohort, a wide variety of courses to support the degree, and an excellent list of faculty mentors and advisors. I successfully applied for acceptance into this program, which I began in September 2006. In 2007, I was awarded a National Library of Medicine F37 informationist fellowship grant to support my graduate studies. After graduating from the CBB program, my title changed to biosciences and bioinformatics librarian.

My involvement with bioinformatics at NUCATS began almost immediately after my hire at Galter in 2006. I met NUBIC's associate director Warren Kibbe to discuss my new position as biosciences librarian and my desire to pursue a master's degree in bioinformatics at Northwestern. After I was accepted to the CBB program, I met NUBIC director Simon Lin at a faculty meet-and-greet poster session for new CBB students. Both NUBIC directors were excited for bioinformatics offerings at the library, and they both agreed to serve on my thesis advisory committee for my CBB degree.

These early meetings led to several years of a good working relationship with bioinformatics at NUCATS and resulted in teaching and publication opportunities for me. On the day I met Simon Lin, I suggested two collaborations to him, prompting him to make a statement that I have quoted many times in talks and posters at conferences over the years: "I love librarians. You connect people to resources, even when the resources are other people" (paraphrased). Librarians as connectors of people is a popular theme in the library world, since the library and librarians are seen as neutral supporters of all faculty and disciplines, and the library's centrality to the institution places librarians in positions to create connections and guide collaboration. This centrality is an important reason that the library can play a key role in CTSA support.

INITIAL PROJECTS WITH NUCATS BIOINFORMATICS UNITS

My first project with NUBIC in 2007 was a very *non*bioinformatics project: usability testing for a Google Gadget Gateway to PubMed (G3P). This project was the brainchild of an undergraduate summer programming intern at NUBIC for Google's Summer of Code project. G3P was a Google Gadget that could be installed on a user's iGoogle page and display results of a user-defined search in the Google home-page interface. It operated on the same basic principle as saving a search and delivering scheduled search results through the My NCBI "Saved Searches" notification system, but the gadget would allow users to see search updates immediately upon opening their iGoogle home page. I was recruited to compose a focus group from different user populations to demonstrate and test G3P and gather focus-group feedback. The focus group included two faculty members (one basic sciences and one clinical), two postdoctoral researchers, two medical students, one basic sciences graduate student, and one statistician. The tool was very well received, but due to changes in PubMed's application program interface (API), production of G3P did not survive beyond one year past the development of the gadget, and the demise of the iGoogle platform ultimately prevented the possibility of reestablishing gadget functionality.

My bioinformatics degree was structured to make me an end-point user-support expert in various bioinformatics techniques rather than training me to become a bioinformatics software developer or algorithm developer. As I became more fluent in bioinformatics techniques and concepts through my coursework, I began to develop my graduate thesis and plans for bioinformatics services and tools to offer, many in close partnership with my mentors at NUCATS. First, I explored the purchase of a site license for Ingenuity Pathway Analysis (IPA) software,[17] to be paid by the library and available to all biomedical researchers at Northwestern University. NUBIC had previously managed a license for IPA, but it was only available for use by the bioinformatics analysts at NUBIC. When Galter Library purchased our license for IPA in 2008, NUBIC was able to drop their license, saving the NUCATS Institute money on licensing fees. Opening up IPA had two other primary benefits: it gave our users the freedom to run their own pathway analyses with IPA, which in turn allowed the analysts at NUBIC to spend more of their time on statistically intensive or specialized computation for users instead of pathway analysis. The license also helped to save our users money; they could utilize IPA for their own analyses and not pay consultant's fees for pathway analysis.

As costs for IPA increased and our acquisitions budget required heavy scrutiny and resource evaluation, we opted to discontinue IPA and chose GeneGo MetaCore (now managed by Thomson Reuters)[18] as the pathway-analysis product to replace IPA in 2010. I recruited two of our pathways' "power users" to test both platforms side by side to compare features and assess overall acceptability of the switch. I then communicated with all of our pathways users, informing them of the reason for the switch, how to migrate their data, and how the change in platform would allow increased simultaneous-user capacity.

During both the licensing of IPA and the subsequent transition to MetaCore, I developed my skills to become a local support expert on the use of both products and also in the use of free pathway platforms such as DAVID (Database for Annotation, Visualization, and Integrated Discovery).[19-21] One project for my CBB degree was a comparison of various pathway-analysis platforms, and the outcome of my expanded facility with these tools enabled my next projects with NUBIC developers: Functional Disease Ontology (FunDO) and GeneAnswers, and a teaching opportunity within a NUCATS master's program.

EXPLORING GENES USING FUNCTIONAL DISEASE ONTOLOGY: FUNDO

FunDO was a network visualization program based on Disease Ontology (DO), an ontology developed by Lynn Schriml of the Institute for Genome Sciences and my advisor Warren Kibbe at NUBIC.[22-25] Disease Ontology semantically links disease phenotypes with putatively causative genes. It was developed to employ text mining to harvest Gene Reference into Function (GeneRIF) data from published literature as depicted in NCBI's gene database[26] to infer gene-disease relationships. When compared to Online Mendelian Inheritance in Man (OMIM),[27] DO displayed better recall of gene-disease relationships and similar precision to OMIM.[24] However, not all potential users of DO were comfortable with using the structured taxonomy browser of DO and preferred a graphical user interface and visual displays of gene-disease relationships. This spurred the creation of FunDO.[23,25] FunDO's code was developed by the same programmer who created G3P, with guidance from NUBIC directors and local DO contributors. To use FunDO, a user pastes a list of genes—such as a list of genes from a microarray experiment—into the interface. FunDO returns a tabular list of all diseases that had GeneRIF annotations to the genes most common among the user's list. The results also included a graph of the top five diseases common in the user's gene list displayed as central nodes with all genes linked to each disease as radially connected nodes. This type of representation made it easy to see genes that are involved in multiple diseases by their gene-disease associations (figure 2.1).

This simple-to-use functionality made FunDO exceedingly popular with users and gave quick answers to users who wished to discover what diseases could be linked to a list of experimental genes. I created a video tutorial on the use of FunDO and wrote news items and a brief guide to its use.[28] FunDO received good reviews from researchers when it was introduced, and they saw it as valuable for a quick investigation into what diseases (besides their disease of interest) could be inferred from the genes from their experiments.

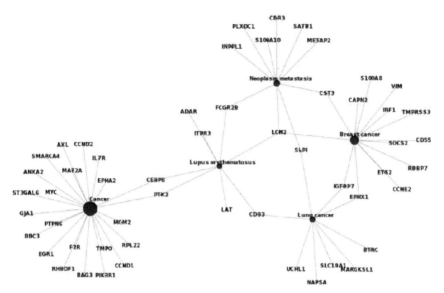

Figure 2.1.   Graph of genes from a Burkitt lymphoma experiment, as interpreted using GeneRIF. Annotations by FunDO.

FunDO was available as an open web-based application and continued to be a popular platform until it was deactivated due to the departure of its developer in the early 2010s. Since then, FunDO's code has not been updated, and a new graphical user interface to Disease Ontology was developed. It is available at http://doa.nubic .northwestern.edu/pages/search.php. However, this interface does not easily facilitate batch loading of gene lists for gene-to-disease interactions, and some disease searches retrieve empty results. Since the deactivation of FunDO, we have discovered that people from all over the world were using FunDO, because I have received many pleas from users asking if it can be reactivated. One of my future goals is to determine if I can resurrect this popular tool.

Additionally, as part of the development of FunDO and for my bioinformatics graduate thesis, I performed a comparison of the functionality of FunDO, DAVID, and IPA to determine what types of inferences could be made from a list of genes, based on the strengths of each platform. Large gene-set analysis often centers on the concept of enrichment: When users compare their list of experimental genes to all known genes in an organism's genome, some genes are heavily represented in functional, disease, or molecular pathways. This overrepresentation of a set of target genes to a specific function, pathway, or process is referred to as enrichment. Enrichment analysis platforms use statistical tests such as Fisher's exact (or hypergeometric) tests to give an estimate of the likelihood that this enrichment is not due to random chance for any given pathway or annotation. Commercial pathway-analysis products use additional algorithms based on causal analysis to extend functional relationships beyond enrichment.[29-31]

Each type of pathway-analysis platform has its own merits: DAVID utilizes numerous sources to deliver lists of enrichment or representation in many categories, such as KEGG[32] canonical pathways, Gene Ontology annotations,[33] or protein functions. Commercial pathway-analysis products use many of these same resources but also develop their own proprietary pathways and functional annotations based on evidence from expert review of biomedical literature by their staff scientists. These commercial pathways and some other web-based or open-source pathway platforms also allow users to include expression values associated with each gene or gene product in their lists.

GENEANSWERS

Similar to FunDO, GeneAnswers is a package for analysis of genotype-phenotype connections, but it is broader in context than FunDO's gene-to-disease limits. GeneAnswers is an R-based package for gene list analysis that can be downloaded from the Bioconductor open-source site.[34] It was created by developers at NUBIC in partnership with developers from the University of Chicago.[35] GeneAnswers utilizes a wide array of other Bioconductor packages to assist users in building visual networks of gene interactions based on a variety of annotation standards, such as Gene Ontology, Disease Ontology, KEGG pathways, Reactome interactions, and other annotations. Users can input a list of genes, with or without experimental values (such as fold changes or measured intensities), and build node and edge diagrams based on their selected set of annotations, heat maps of gene-concept cross-tabulations, or tabular results of enrichment tests. My role in this project was very similar to my role in supporting FunDO: I was asked to run comparison analyses in GeneAnswers, DAVID, and MetaCore. This comparison led to my inclusion as a coauthor on a publication describing GeneAnswers.[36]

TEACHING PATHWAY ANALYSIS TO MSCI STUDENTS

A new opportunity for me came as a result came of the comparison I did among DAVID, IPA, and FunDO and the support I provide for users of MetaCore: I was asked to be a guest lecturer in the bioinformatics course for our CTS institute's master of science in clinical investigation (MSCI).[37] MSCI programs aim to train medical practitioners in skills necessary for research and publication—skills they may not have developed during their training as medical students or residents. The coursework includes classes in topics such as grantsmanship, team science, epidemiology and statistics, clinical trials design, drug development, and bioinformatics (often as an elective). I was invited to teach a module on pathway analysis for our MSCI bioinformatics course. I concentrated on inference of function from gene sets and discovery of biomarkers for disease using current databases and tools, and I was asked by the course director to highlight MetaCore, DAVID, and FunDO.

Teaching MSCI students is challenging: Some of these students are many years removed from classes in molecular biology, so I had to create ways to make pathway inference relevant and interesting to a largely clinical audience. One student even asked me, "How is any of this relevant to clinical practice?" My response was that some diseases share a surprising number of common genes. Some of these shared genes are simply genes that are required for normal biological processes so are common among normal functioning and pathological conditions alike, but other shared genes can provide insight into aberrant processes or functional connections between seemingly unrelated diseases. These connections help to provide new avenues for treating diseases that were not originally considered before these common biomarker links were found.

Some classroom examples I provided included the connections between viruses and certain types of cancer or connections between inflammatory markers and Alzheimer's disease. Once we generated pathway maps and discovered process linkages among common genes, the value of this type of analysis became more relevant to the students. This discovery of the research potential for new uses for existing drugs or novel experimental avenues had meaning for them. I also emphasized the fact that commercial pathway-analysis platforms and GeneRIF annotations provide links to published literature evidence used to support inferred network interactions. I've always considered this expert manual curation of literature in pathway analysis to be an extension of evidence-based medicine (EBM) but in a more molecular context. This EBM-like feature of some pathway platforms was appreciated by the students.

As mentioned earlier, GeneGo MetaCore was the commercial pathway platform we used for the class, and the students found its network-building options overwhelming at first. Simply importing a list of genes into the software's input interface and clicking "build network" results in confusing diagrams of interactions. The students soon realized that if they formulated a hypothesis to pursue regarding their gene lists, they could develop more meaningful and focused network diagrams. They discovered that they could focus their networks on gene function in specific tissues, or build networks based on activation or inhibition of target genes. This type of critical thinking is necessary in pathway analysis, and it is always satisfying for me to observe users developing their analytical skills when working with these packages. Students in the class found FunDO to be much simpler to use overall than either DAVID or MetaCore because it concentrated only on disease-gene relationships, so decisions based on molecular function or processes were not necessary. However, they realized that beyond the disease-gene relationships, FunDO did not give them information upon which to build hypotheses based on biological function, such as cellular responses to stress, programmed cell death, and other more global processes implicated in disease. The more complicated results returned by DAVID and MetaCore took a little more time to interpret by the students, but many of them found this discovery of complex functional interactivity to be incredibly fascinating, and it opened their eyes to new sources of evidence for gene-disease relationships.

At this time, I am no longer a guest instructor for the MSCI bioinformatics class due to the departure of the instructor who solicited my expertise, but my increased interaction with NUCATS since our integration into the institute is providing promising new collaboration opportunities, and I hope to once again contribute to curriculum-based instruction. For the present, I am working on seminar and workshop series, organized with NUCATS instructors and hosted by the library.

BIOINFORMATICS SUPPORT FROM THE LIBRARY: TEACHING, TRAINING, AND TRANSLATION

In addition to the projects mentioned above, I have developed a number of guides and library-based workshops on mostly open-source or web-based bioinformatics tools and databases, such as the NCBI suite of databases, the European Bioinformatics (EBI) database suite, the UCSC (University California, Santa Cruz) Genome Browser, and several more. These workshops were developed as a goal and capstone of my completion of my bioinformatics degree. They are available by request to our user community, and I offer the most popular workshops (particularly the UCSC Genome Browser session) at least a couple of times a year. These workshops are not specifically designed for support of our CTS institute or translational research, but much of biomedical research is translational by nature, so I find that my sessions and consultations still support the translational research enterprise, even if they are not specifically labeled as translational. Some of my greatest feelings of satisfaction have come from the attendance of some of our CTSA faculty and researchers at my workshops and having them tell me that they have taken away knowledge on the use of these resources that they never had before.

NIH funding for individual research grants (R01s) is limited, and competition for these grants is heavy,[38,39] so investigators are under pressure to prove the relevance of their basic science project grants to impact the advancement of health outcomes. This is the nature of the translational science continuum: to speed the "translation" of basic science or molecular level discoveries to therapies and overall population health improvement.[40–42] The translational continuum is also not unidirectional: Clinical observations of disease will often inform new molecular or animal models of treatment, taking the "bedside" back to the "bench."[43] Not all universities have CTS grants, though many medical schools have some type of translational science institute or support for team-based science. Librarians with bioinformatics training can provide context and meaning for clinicians by highlighting the genomic basis of disease, and medical librarians of all backgrounds help excavate evidence for translational research from bench to bedside to population health. Translational researchers do not have the time to investigate all of the informatics resources that are available to them or to conduct thorough searches of literature to support their research, so the role of the librarian supporting translational science is more valuable than ever.

Molecular interactions are never simple, even to experts in biochemistry or molecular biology. Because most investigators work in highly focused and sometimes narrow topics of biomedicine, it is very rare that any single scientist has a comprehensive knowledge of all functional interactions among genes or biomolecules. Instructing users in the selection and application of bioinformatics tools is, in many ways, similar to conducting a good reference interview: the user must be guided to formulate a directed hypothesis for which they are seeking evidence. Sometimes I'll begin a consultation with a user who says, "I need to use [this tool]," but after I ask them questions about what they want to know, we realize that a different tool or set of tools is more appropriate for their question. Any information source is a tool, and the question for investigation should dominate the tool selection rather than the tool dominating the investigation.

Library-based bioinformatics experts do not need to be experts in all fields of genetics or molecular biology but instead must understand the purpose and strengths of the tools or databases they support in order to guide users to the best tools for their research. Sometimes this process requires testing and using multiple tools; I find that our users don't have the time or expertise to investigate which tools are best for each intended purpose. This is how I have made myself valuable to our CTS institute's bioinformatics group: I can help users explore questions that can be answered using current tools and databases available to us. If none of these options suit their needs, they can contract the bioinformatics and biostatistics analysts at NUCATS to perform specialized or complex analyses on their data. Additionally, I have an excellent working relationship with our Next-Generation Sequencing Core (NGS Core). This core provides free consultation to medical school researchers and performs complex analyses on a fee-for-service basis. My relationship with the director of the core has allowed me to develop an understanding of the sources of support I can recommend to our users when their needs go beyond my own skills in consultation and instruction.

CURRENT AND FUTURE PROJECTS

My involvement with NUCATS goes well beyond bioinformatics support, and I have contributed to numerous projects and initiatives, especially in support of our most recent CTSA proposal. I have assisted NUCATS in linking the CTS award with publications using My NCBI, led the library efforts to track T-scholars publications for NUCATS T-grant mentors, and contributed to team science efforts for NUCATS. Increasing awareness of bioinformatics support from Galter Library has been my goal for several years. It has been made easier by our integration with NUCATS and an emphasis by our new director on informatics, which has helped me progress my bioinformatics support goals more rapidly than I could on my own.

At the time this chapter is being written, my current and future plans for bioinformatics projects in the library for our translational researchers and the medical campus at large include a seminar series entitled "Computational Skills for Informatics," featuring guest speakers from our university research computing group, a biostatistics faculty member, and our NGS Core director. Topics include cloud computing, NGS techniques, best practices, and a discussion on reproducible research. I am already beginning to develop ideas for another series of guest seminars on more topics of this nature.

I have also begun scheduling extended-format workshops to be hosted by the library. We will be hosting a Galaxy project[44] trainer for a daylong, hands-on workshop in the use of the Galaxy web-based genomics and sequence-methods software platform. Additionally, I have begun discussions with local experts for other extended format "boot camp" topics on R scripting, Python scripting, and NGS techniques.

Recently, Galter Library utilized a onetime budget allotment to purchase six new research computers, which we equipped with a number of new informatics and statistical software packages including Vector NTI,[39] DNASTAR Lasergene,[40] Atlas.ti,[41] GraphPad Prism,[42] Golden Helix SNP and Variation Suite[43] (installed on one computer), Partek Genomics Suite[44] (installed on one computer), and a number of statistical packages. This solution of purchasing stand-alone or "kiosk" licenses for multiple years allowed us to purchase a wider variety and number of informatics packages than we could if we had attempted to purchase dynamic site licenses for user download or online software use. Bioinformatics resources can be expensive, and we don't have a guarantee of an extended budget for site licenses, so the computer research station was our best solution—and it encourages users to come to the library to use the software and perhaps learn more about our staff and other services while they're here.

SUCCESSES AND CHALLENGES

Overall, I would say that my experiences in partnering with our CTSA for bioinformatics projects and support have been very successful and positive. Each of my projects helped set the stage for the next one, and my partnerships progressed step by step with NUCATS. I have had a few "slow periods" when fewer opportunities or viable collaborations were available, but I am optimistic for the future.

I would say that the greatest catalyst for successful collaboration has been my partnerships made at the CTS institute among the bioinformatics and biostatistics teams. Some of these partners were introduced to me through my graduate work in bioinformatics and others I have met through shared colleague introductions and at medical school events such as Research Day. We all know this to be true: Some of our best collaborations can arise from a serendipitous meeting at a poster session or in a hallway encounter.

Other important partnerships have helped me develop our teaching and seminar programs. My partnership with our university research computing staff grew out of my role as cochair of Northwestern's E-Science Working Group and has resulted in our computational skills seminar series, and my delegation as Northwestern's NIH Public Access Policy Monitor Role (PACR) has raised my profile in our Office for Sponsored Research, which has led to new opportunities for partnership on data-management policy and data use agreement education for our user community.

Setbacks or challenges to my goals and projects have come in the form of the departure of some of these key partners: Two of my former thesis advisors from NUBIC left the university for other institutions, and this resulted in the loss of my teaching opportunity for the MSCI bioinformatics course. Bioinformatics support at our CTS institute has undergone a few changes in structure and leadership over the past few years, but it has always developed excellent tools and projects; my regret is that not all of these projects have been sustained (such as FunDO). My hope is that our recent integration with NUCATS will lead to more collaboration opportunities on projects in the future, and this does seem to be likely because NUCATS informatics leadership is enthusiastic and encouraging of Galter participation.

My advice to other library-based informatics experts is not very novel, and I've heard these words from many other librarians when discussing support of CTSA partners: "Get out there!" In some ways, my long history at Northwestern may be my best asset, because every year here increases my professional network, but active participation in a variety of campus research events can substitute for institutional longevity for newly hired CTSA support librarians. Attending events such as the Research Day poster sessions or departmental seminars has opened lots of doors for me and given me new ideas to bring home to my work in the library. Finding one or two knowledgeable and action-oriented partners is also invaluable. These partners can be within the library, such as the highly supportive director or associate director who sings your praises to CTS leadership, or outside the library, such as the core facility director with whom you chatted at a campus event who knows the ins and outs of university leadership and policy, or a faculty member with whom you have consulted on a large project resulting in publication.

In the past my largest stumbling block was my concern that I didn't have enough expertise to stand among our research community. Then I realized I didn't have to know all the answers or how to do everything myself. I just have to know where to find the answers and the right resources, even when those resources are other people.

NOTES

1. About Northwestern: History. http://www.northwestern.edu/about/facts/history.html. Accessed January 12, 2015.

2. History of Northwestern University Feinberg School of Medicine. http://www.feinberg.northwestern.edu/docs/Feinberg-history-narrative2.pdf. Accessed January 12, 2015.

3. Galter Health Sciences Library: About us; History of the library. 2013. http://www.galter.northwestern.edu/about-us/history-of-the-library. Accessed January 12, 2015.

4. About NUCATS. http://www.nucats.northwestern.edu/about. Accessed January 12, 2015.

5. Lyon J, Giuse NB, Williams A, Koonce T, Walden R. A model for training the new bioinformationist. *J Med Libr Assoc.* 2004;92(2):188–95.

6. Helms AJ, Bradford KD, Warren NJ, Schwartz DG. Bioinformatics opportunities for health sciences librarians and information professionals. *J Med Libr Assoc.* 2004;92(4):489–93.

7. Tennant MR. Bioinformatics librarian: Meeting the information needs of genetics and bioinformatics researchers. *Ref Serv Rev.* 2005;33(1):12–19.

8. Chattopadhyay A, Tannery NH, Silverman DAL, Bergen P, Epstein BA. Design and implementation of a library-based information service in molecular biology and genetics at the University of Pittsburgh. *J Med Libr Assoc.* 2006;94(3):307–13,E192.

9. Geer RC, Rein DC. Building the role of medical libraries in bioinformatics. *J Med Libr Assoc.* 2006;94(3):284–85.

10. Geer RC. Broad issues to consider for library involvement in bioinformatics. *J Med Libr Assoc.* 2006;94(3):286–98,E152–55.

11. Lyon JA, Tennant MR, Messner KR, Osterbur DL. Carving a niche: Establishing bioinformatics collaborations. *J Med Libr Assoc.* 2006;94(3):330–35.

12. Minie M, Bowers S, Tarczy-Hornoch P, et al. The University of Washington Health Sciences Library BioCommons: An evolving Northwest biomedical research information support infrastructure. *J Med Libr Assoc.* 2006;94(3):321–29.

13. Osterbur DL, Alpi K, Canevari C, et al. Vignettes: Diverse library staff offering diverse bioinformatics services. *J Med Libr Assoc.* 2006;94(3):306,E388–91.

14. Rein DC. Developing library bioinformatics services in context: The Purdue University Libraries bioinformationist program. *J Med Libr Assoc.* 2006;94(3):314–20,E193–97.

15. Tennant MR, Miyamoto MM. The role of the medical librarian in the basic biological sciences: A case study in virology and evolution. *J Med Libr Assoc.* 2008;96(4):290–98.

16. Li M, Chen YB, Clintworth WA. Expanding roles in a library-based bioinformatics service program: A case study. *J Med Libr Assoc.* 2013;101(4):303–9.

17. Ingenuity Pathway Analysis website. http://www.ingenuity.com/products/ipa. Accessed January 12, 2015.

18. MetaCore. http://thomsonreuters.com/metacore. Accessed January 12, 2015.

19. Huang da W, Sherman BT, Lempicki RA. Systematic and integrative analysis of large gene lists using DAVID bioinformatics resources. *Nat Protoc.* 2009;4(1):44–57.

20. Huang da W, Sherman BT, Stephens R, Baseler MW, Lane HC, Lempicki RA. DAVID gene ID conversion tool. *Bioinformation.* 2008;2(10):428–30.

21. Dennis G, Jr., Sherman BT, Hosack DA, et al. DAVID: Database for Annotation, Visualization, and Integrated Discovery. *Genome Biology.* 2003;4(5):P3.

22. Kibbe WA, Arze C, Felix V, et al. Disease Ontology 2015 update: An expanded and updated database of human diseases for linking biomedical knowledge through disease data. *Nucleic Acids Res.* 2014;43(D1):D1071–78.

23. Schriml LM, Arze C, Nadendla S, et al. Disease Ontology: A backbone for disease semantic integration. *Nucleic Acids Res.* 2012;40(Database issue):D940–46.

24. Osborne JD, Flatow J, Holko M, et al. Annotating the human genome with Disease Ontology. *BMC Genomics.* 2009;10 Suppl 1:S6.

25. Du P, Feng G, Flatow J, et al. From Disease Ontology to disease-ontology lite: Statistical methods to adapt a general-purpose ontology for the test of gene-ontology associations. *Bioinformatics.* 2009;25(12):i63–68.

26. National Center for Biotechnology Information (NCBI). GeneRIF: Gene Reference into Function. 2014. http://www.ncbi.nlm.nih.gov/gene/about-generif. Accessed January 12, 2015.

27. McKusick-Nathans Institute of Genetic Medicine. Online Mendelian Inheritance in Man, OMIM®. http://www.omim.org/. Accessed January 17, 2015.

28. Shaw PL. Functional Disease Ontology (FunDO). 2009. http://www.galter.northwestern.edu/guides-and-tutorials/functional-disease-ontology. Accessed January 12, 2015.

29. IPA Network Generation Algorithm (white paper). 2005. http://www.ingenuity.com/wp-content/themes/ingenuity-qiagen/pdf/ipa/IPA-netgen-algorithm-whitepaper.pdf.

30. Kramer A, Green J, Pollard J, Jr., Tugendreich S. Causal analysis approaches in Ingenuity Pathway Analysis. *Bioinformatics*. 2014;30(4):523–30.

31. Ekins S, Bugrim A, Brovold L, et al. White Paper: Algorithms for Network Analysis. 2014.

32. Ogata H, Goto S, Sato K, Fujibuchi W, Bono H, Kanehisa M. KEGG: Kyoto Encyclopedia of Genes and Genomes. *Nucleic Acids Res*. 1999;27(1):29–34.

33. Ashburner M, Ball CA, Blake JA, et al. Gene ontology: Tool for the unification of biology. Gene Ontology Consortium. *Nat Genet*. 2000;25(1):25–29.

34. Bioconductor: Open-source software for bioinformatics. 2003. http://bioconductor.org/. Accessed January 22, 2015.

35. Feng G, Du P, Krett NL, et al. A collection of Bioconductor methods to visualize gene-list annotations. *BMC Research Notes*. 2010;3:10.

36. Feng G, Shaw P, Rosen ST, Lin SM, Kibbe WA. Using the Bioconductor GeneAnswers package to interpret gene lists. *Meth Mol Bio*. 2012;802:101–12.

37. Northwestern University, NUCATS. Master of science in clinical investigation (MSCI). http://www.nucats.northwestern.edu/education-career-development/graduate-programs/master-science-clinical-investigation-msci. Accessed January 12, 2015.

38. Rockey S. Comparing success rates, award rates, and funding rates. *Rock Talk*. 2014. http://nexus.od.nih.gov/all/2014/03/05/comparing-success-award-funding-rates. Accessed April 15, 2015.

39. Rockey S. Application success rates decline in 2013. *Rock Talk*. 2014. http://nexus.od.nih.gov/all/2013/12/18/application-success-rates-decline-in-2013. Accessed April 15, 2015.

40. Sung NS, Crowley WF, Jr., Genel M, et al. Central challenges facing the national clinical research enterprise. *JAMA*. 2003;289(10):1278–87.

41. Dougherty D, Conway PH. The "3T's" road map to transform US health care: The "how" of high-quality care. *JAMA*. 2008;299(19):2319–21.

42. Drolet BC, Lorenzi NM. Translational research: Understanding the continuum from bench to bedside. *Transl Res*. 2011;157(1):1–5.

43. Rubio DM, Schoenbaum EE, Lee LS, et al. Defining translational research: Implications for training. *Acad Med*. 2010;85(3):470–75.

44. The Galaxy Project. http://galaxyproject.org/. Accessed January 21, 2015.

3

Librarian Involvement in tranSMART

A Translational Biomedical Research Platform

Marci D. Brandenburg

INTRODUCTION

This is the story of collaboration between a librarian, her university, and an international community focused on using, developing, and advancing a translational biomedical research platform called tranSMART. TranSMART is a data-sharing and analysis platform developed by a pharmaceutical company that has grown to include academia, noncommercial groups, and international partners to provide an open-source knowledge-management platform. As a librarian at one of the main academic partners, I became a key member of the tranSMART community by providing training, documentation, evaluations, and other vital contributions.

BACKGROUND

Founded in 1817, the University of Michigan (U-M) is a public research university located in Ann Arbor, Michigan. U-M consists of nineteen schools and colleges and has an enrollment of approximately 43,700 undergraduate, graduate, and professional students. The U-M Medical School was founded in 1850, graduates approximately 170 physicians each year, and receives close to 70 percent of the funds awarded by the National Institutes of Health (NIH) to the entire university.[1] The medical school consists of twenty clinical departments and nine basic science departments. U-M has invested greatly in translational research and provides a home to multiple centers and groups focused on all stages of bench-to-bedside research.

In 2005, the U-M founded the National Center for Integrative Biomedical Informatics (NCIBI, http://www.ncibi.org/) as one of the NIH's National Centers for Biomedical Computing[2] and created the Center for Computational Medicine and Bioinformatics (CCMB, http://www.ccmb.med.umich.edu/ccmb), a campus-wide interdisciplinary center with more than one hundred affiliated faculty members. The Michigan Institute for Clinical and Health Research (MICHR, http://www.michr. umich.edu/home), which is a member of the Clinical and Translational Science Award (CTSA) consortium, was established in 2006. In 2012, the U-M Medical School created the Department of Computational Medicine and Bioinformatics (DCM&B, http://www.ccmb.med.umich.edu/) with the mission of "training the next generation of innovators and leaders in this field, applying to create new science, translational research, and creating new methods to improve public health and societal welfare."[3] The U-M bioinformatics graduate program, CCMB, and NCIBI are all now housed within DCM&B.

The Taubman Health Sciences Library (THL), a unit of the larger U-M Library System, provides services to and collaborates with faculty, staff, and students in all the health sciences departments, schools, colleges, and centers, including those areas engaged in clinical and translational science. In 2005, THL partnered with NCIBI to create a pilot bioinformationist position. The success of this pilot ultimately led to my hiring in November 2010 as a permanent, full-time bioinformationist.

As THL's bioinformationist, I provide information services to bioinformatics researchers on campus. The National Library of Medicine (NLM) has defined informationists as "information specialists who have received graduate training and practical experience that provides them with disciplinary background both in biomedical, behavioral or biological sciences and information sciences/informatics."[4] In addition to majoring in biology and environmental studies in college, I have an MS in biology and an MS in information. As the bioinformationist, I work closely with the U-M faculty and staff in the field of bioinformatics. I offer workshops and develop instructional resources for several locally developed bioinformatics tools, organize the programming for a weekly seminar series, attend a bioinformatics journal club, and more. Although my home department is in THL, I am fully embedded in the DCM&B and the medical school's Bioinformatics Core, a for-fee bioinformatics analysis unit, and both pay a portion of my salary. As a result, I am intimately involved in initiatives taken on by these groups, including work involving tranSMART.

TRANSMART

The tranSMART platform was originally developed by Johnson & Johnson and Recombinant Data Corporation as a data-management system for Johnson & Johnson's pharmaceutical researchers, and it became open-source in 2013. U-M is a founding member of the tranSMART Foundation (http://transmartfoundation.org/), a nonprofit organization that serves as the community home for the tranSMART platform.[5]

**Table 3.1. Member/partner institutions of the tranSMART
Foundation, including institution type, as of April 28, 2015**

Member	Type of Institution
ConvergeHEALTH by Deloitte	Commercial
Johns Hopkins University	Academic
Oracle	Commercial
PerkinElmer	Commercial
Pfizer	Commercial
Roche	Commercial
Sanofi	Commercial
Takeda	Commercial
University of Michigan	Academic
ARLION	Commercial
AssureRx	Commercial
Cognizant	Commercial
DExStR	Commercial
The Hyve	Commercial
Institute for Systems Biology	Nonprofit
IO Informatics	Commercial
One Mind	Nonprofit
Philips	Commercial
BT-GS	Commercial
Elevada	Commercial
Harvard University	Academic
Rancho Biosciences	Commercial

Founded in 2013, the tranSMART Foundation is made up of nonprofit organizations, commercial entities, and academic institutions. In addition to the U-M, examples of other foundation members include Johns Hopkins University, Oracle, Sanofi, ConvergeHEALTH by Deloitte, the Hyve, One Mind, and Harvard University (table 3.1). The mission of the foundation is to enable "effective sharing, integration, standardization and analysis of heterogeneous data from collaborative translational research by mobilizing the tranSMART open-source and open-data community."[6]

The tranSMART platform provides access to data and analysis tools; both private and publicly available data sets can be loaded into the platform. Although there is a web-based demonstration version of tranSMART with preloaded, publicly available data, the platform is meant to be installed on a local server. When the platform is initially installed, it contains no preloaded data and will need to be populated with private and publicly available data sets. Clinical demographic data, such as race, age, and sex, can be loaded for each sample, in addition to survival time, disease or study categories, gene expression data, and more. One strength of tranSMART is its ability to integrate such a wide variety of data types. A cross-platform analysis of cohorts can then be performed; for example, one could look at the survival time in years of women with breast cancer under fifty years of age compared to women over fifty years of age.

TranSMART provides the translational research community with an open-source platform that allows for easy sharing, access, and analysis of large amounts of data, both molecular and clinical. It facilitates hypothesis generation and testing, and uses a role-based security model to ensure security and privacy of research data.[7] Comparable translational resources include BRISK (Biology-Related Information Storage Kit; a data integration and management platform originally designed to improve data sharing and collaboration), iDASH (Integrating Data for Analysis, Anonymization, and SHaring; provides tools for data sharing and analysis), cBioPortal for Cancer Genomics (provides tools to visualize, analyze, and access genomics data sets), and iCOD Portal (Integrated Clinical Omics Database; provides means to view and analyze molecular data combined with disease information).[8] There are plans to connect tranSMART to REDCap (a secure application for building and managing surveys and databases), and work has been done to integrate it with high-performing data-analysis software, such as Genedata Analyst.[9]

My involvement with tranSMART began when the chair of DCM&B, who is very familiar with my skills and expertise, asked me to participate in U-M's role as a tranSMART member. I joined a local U-M tranSMART team made up of DCM&B faculty and staff. I have provided instruction and instructional resources on using tranSMART, participated in the tranSMART community, and assessed tranSMART for use by U-M researchers. My work on the tranSMART project strengthened my relationship with many local collaborators and introduced me to additional national and international collaborators. The rest of the chapter will describe my role in instruction-related activities, project management, mentorship, tool evaluation, and the tranSMART community.

INSTRUCTION-RELATED ACTIVITIES

As a bioinformationist, I design and conduct numerous instructional activities for locally developed resources. My experience providing hands-on workshops, developing video tutorials, and updating user manuals for these resources laid the groundwork for my involvement with tranSMART. My role in training is highly useful as increased adoption of this translational research platform would lead to further advances in translational research, due to its data-sharing capabilities and fostering of a collaborative environment. The creation of documentation and training to accelerate learning for new users is a key factor to quicker acceptance and adoption of the tranSMART platform.

User Guides

The University of Michigan's involvement with tranSMART began in 2012, prior to both the establishment of the tranSMART Foundation and the release of the open-source version of the platform, version 1.1. At that time the tranSMART community was relatively small, consisting of approximately forty individuals. In 2011 and 2012, Recombinant (now ConvergeHEALTH by Deloitte) created a tranSMART user's guide and user administration guide for tranSMART version 1.0. The user's guide is a one-hundred-plus-page document that introduces the end user to the interface and provides step-by-step instructions for running advanced analyses. The user administration guide is an approximately thirty-page document that covers the responsibilities of administrators, such as creating new user accounts and granting appropriate levels of access. In 2013, it was necessary to update these manuals for the release of tranSMART version 1.1.

The chair of DCM&B asked me to be part of a local documentation team charged with updating these manuals in time for the new release. The team included DCM&B programmers who write computer code to develop or improve software programs and who had been working on tranSMART. At that time my familiarity with tranSMART was limited, so my first step was to do a hands-on walk-through with the existing user guide and the soon-to-be-released version 1.1 of the platform. I noted all areas of discrepancy between the manual and the current interface. I then updated necessary screenshots and text in the manual to match the current interface. I used the same process for the administration guide. Next, I shared the changes with the local documentation team, which made additional changes and edits as needed. The updated guides were made available under a Creative Commons (CC) Attribution 3.0 Unported license with the release of tranSMART version 1.1 in September 2013. This license allows individuals to share and adapt these resources for any purpose, including commercial use, as long as attribution is provided.[10] The value of using this CC license is that tranSMART users can manipulate the guides to meet their own needs, allowing for the creation of detailed training resources and easier updating for future software version releases.

Understanding the currently loaded data in tranSMART was a major challenge I encountered at this stage in the project. Once a group adopts the tranSMART platform, they install their own version that is then shared with their individual collaborators. Although there is now a publicly available demonstration version of tranSMART that can be used for basic exploration of the platform, at this phase in the project there was no such version accessible to everyone. As no publicly available demonstration version existed, the tranSMART version I accessed did not have the same data as the version used in the original user guide. As a result, trial and error was required to determine what data and data types were necessary for various analyses. This also meant that I was unable to run certain analyses as I did not have access to the appropriate data. For example, if an analysis required two data variables in numerical format, but my data set only had one numerical data variable, then I was incapable of performing this analysis and couldn't write or update the requisite documentation.

Being part of a team was extremely beneficial, as I was able to work with the programmers to better understand the interface and update the documentation in a timely manner. All members of the local documentation team were relatively new to tranSMART; this resulted in knowledge gaps in how to use certain tranSMART features. Learning the full range of this platform's capabilities proved to be a group effort; this reinforced my association with members of the local tranSMART team. One notable benefit of this work was that it strengthened my relationships with the DCM&B programmers. This proved to be valuable since my tranSMART involvement continued beyond this initial documentation project.

Additionally, my role in this documentation project provided me with a hands-on opportunity to learn more about the platform and to investigate its features and functionality; this drastically increased my knowledge of tranSMART. Going through the process of documenting step-by-step instructions for using a resource is one of the best ways to learn a new tool. Librarians are accustomed to providing step-by-step instructions for accessing library resources, so we understand the level of detail that is beneficial in user guides. Therefore, the transition to writing software user guides is a natural one, and the knowledge gained during guide creation can be applied to other forms of training on the resource. Providing these user guides gives the tranSMART community current resources for learning the tool and can increase its adoption.

Video Tutorials

In December 2012, I worked with the director of informatics infrastructure in DCM&B to facilitate three project proposals involving a total of nine faculty members as part of an internal U-M interdisciplinary funding opportunity. Due to funding requirements, three faculty members were required for a successful submission, but the same faculty member could not be named on multiple proposals. Funding of the proposals was determined by a random process, and the use of the majority of the funds was limited to student and postdoctoral candidate salaries. I was a named faculty member on one of the proposals along with a faculty member from DCM&B and one from internal medicine. Although my proposal did not ultimately get funded, the other two tranSMART projects did receive funding. My role in the formation and submission, including identifying relevant faculty, was significant, as was my role in carrying out the funded work.

My involvement in the two funded projects was crucial to their success; I provided leadership, facilitated project management, and mentored the students throughout the process. When we received notification of funding, stakeholders met several times to determine project objectives and discuss student recruitment. I attended these meetings, wrote multiple job descriptions, and hired students to work on different areas of the projects. Hiring two students to work on the same project provided an additional element of teamwork and made my job easier because the students could rely on each other in addition to me. During the hiring process, I often looked for complementary skills and backgrounds; this presented additional opportunities for the students to learn from each other.

Throughout the projects, I hired and mentored four students, two of whom worked on tranSMART instruction resources and two of whom did an assessment project. In addition, I was closely involved with the hiring and work of three additional students. Two graduate students, one from U-M's biomedical engineering department and one from the U-M School of Information, were hired in January 2014 to develop tranSMART instructional resources. I was their primary mentor and supervisor and provided them with guidance and support.

Our initial tasks stemmed from my interactions with a DCM&B programmer; after talking with him, I learned of a need for documentation on the tranSMART data-loading process. Given that data loading was often a confusing and frustrating process for potential users, the lack of instructional resources was a significant concern. As increasing adoption and use of tranSMART was one of the primary goals, filling this gap in documentation was my first priority.

When my students began this project, neither had any experience with tranSMART, so the first step for them was to become familiar with the tranSMART platform, followed by the data-loading process. I introduced them to the platform and directed them to existing user manuals and recorded presentations. As I believed a team-based approach would be most meaningful for the students, I encouraged them to work together and scheduled meetings with appropriate collaborators. For example, two other students were working on loading data into tranSMART under the mentorship of a DCM&B programmer. I facilitated a meeting between the four students so that the data loaders could teach the data-loading process to the documentation students. This provided a more collaborative atmosphere for the students, enhancing their experience. This team-based approach was a successful strategy that I hope to implement in future mentoring opportunities.

The documentation team students and I agreed that providing data-loading instructions in multiple teaching formats would be ideal to create learning opportunities to meet a variety of user needs. Video tutorials provide an on-demand means for learning how to use a resource. Different people learn in different ways as some learn better visually, while others prefer reading text or hearing information. To target all types of learning, it is valuable to have video tutorials in addition to written user guides. As a result, both a data-loading manual and a video tutorial were created. I encouraged the students to research screen-capture and video-editing software to determine the best fit for our needs. We considered cost and features such as ease of use and editing capability before ultimately deciding to use Camtasia.

To increase efficiency and productivity, yet maintain a collaborative environment, one student was tasked with working on the data-loading manual, while the other student worked on the data-loading video tutorial. The students decided between themselves who would work on which format, based on their past experiences and future interests. This separation of responsibility meant that each student had an independent assignment, yet they were collectively involved in creating instructional resources on the same topic, data loading. Both students could focus their efforts

Table 3.2. List of tranSMART video tutorials and other training materials created under my mentorship

Video Tutorials	Other Instructional Materials
Data loading • Setting up data-loading client for Mac • Creating a new study and loading clinical data	Written user manual • Clinical data-loading guide
Advanced analyses • Box plot with ANOVA • Heatmaps (covers four types of heatmaps) • Principal component analysis • Scatter plot with linear regression • Table with Fisher test	Hands-on workshop • Introduction to tranSMART (July 2014)
Other • Creating gene signatures • Interface differences between version 1.1 and version 1.2	

while providing feedback on each other's product. I also reviewed and provided feedback on the video tutorial script and video drafts, in addition to the written user manual. The near-final products were shared with the data-loading students and their supervising DCM&B programmer for feedback.

Once the data-loading documents were completed, we moved onto creating video tutorials on how to run a series of advanced analyses using the tranSMART platform, in addition to other tranSMART features. In all, nine video tutorials and one written manual were created under my mentorship (table 3.2). All video tutorials included closed captioning to make the videos more accessible to individuals with disabilities.

Once the video tutorials were completed, I shared them with stakeholders at U-M, including DCM&B programmers and the chair of DCM&B. In addition, I connected with the tranSMART Foundation's vice president of marketing to have all video tutorials hosted on the Foundation's YouTube channel (https://www.youtube.com/playlist?list=PLv0yMFogDiDhBc_nOoHkCwCGY_Fu8hK6D). This afforded me an excellent opportunity to interact with a newer member of the tranSMART Foundation's management team, increasing my visibility. Finally, I uploaded the data-loading manual to the tranSMART Foundation's wiki. As a result, all of these instruction materials are freely available to the worldwide tranSMART community, helping current and potential users navigate the tranSMART platform.

Since the creation of these materials, I have received questions related to the training resources from a London solution manager for a research and development software company and from a nonprofit neuroinformatics organization in Sweden. In addition, collaborators at U-M and Johns Hopkins University have informed me that they have viewed the tutorials and found them useful. Additionally, in response to these instruction materials, a collaborator from a scientific data consulting company wrote, "You are a rock star—wow! This is amazing. I don't think the community is aware of all these rich resources."

From the beginning, we were faced with a difficult decision regarding the development of these instruction materials. We knew that a newer version of tranSMART, tranSMART version 1.2, would be released in the near future. Since only version 1.1 was available to us at the time, our options were to create tutorials on version 1.1 or create nothing until the new version was released (which was not really an option since the student funding would no longer be available!). Knowing this, we attempted to address topics that would translate easily to the new version, ensuring that the videos would remain relevant and useful even with newer versions of the software and possible interface changes. For example, I knew that version 1.1's advanced analyses capabilities would still exist in the new version and that the process for running them would be similar. In version 1.2, released in August 2014, the interface changed slightly, moving the advanced analyses to a different tab, but the capabilities remained the same. Although our video tutorials display an earlier version of the interface, they demonstrate identical functions; therefore, despite the release of a newer version, I believe these tutorials still have value for users of previous versions. As of April 2015 most of our tutorials had been viewed more than 150 times, with more than half being viewed more than 250 times. The last video tutorial we created has been the most popular with more than 420 views; this video shows interface changes between version 1.1 and version 1.2.

I attribute the success of these projects to several factors. First, I believe my work with the students was essential to our success. I provided a flexible work environment for the students, leaving them free to work at times and locations that were convenient for them. The students really appreciated this flexibility as it helped them better manage their tight and irregular schedules, constrained by classes, assignments, and other obligations. This flexible environment decreased the likelihood of school and work conflicts, increased student satisfaction, and expanded the amount of time and effort they could put toward these projects. To keep things on track, I held weekly in-person meetings to ensure that we remained on schedule with the creation of instruction resources. At these meetings, the students asked me questions, we made group decisions about the look and feel of the videos, we divvied up responsibilities, and more. In between meetings, the students shared drafts of their work, and I provided feedback to ensure that their work was both pertinent and productive.

Good project-management skills were also essential to success, since each project involved multiple people and numerous deliverables. To enhance teamwork and productivity, I met weekly with the students, as previously described. These meetings kept the project on track and gave us an opportunity to regularly discuss issues, concerns, and progress. We used Google Drive to share drafts and final products, helping us manage version control and the sharing of large video files. The knowledge acquired during the creation of these materials allowed us to offer another type of learning opportunity—hands-on training sessions.

Hands-On Training Sessions

Although many of the bioinformatics instruction sessions I offer at U-M are open for anyone to attend, I am occasionally asked to teach a curriculum-based session. One day, during a conversation with a DCM&B faculty member, I suggested covering tranSMART in his class. As a result, in April 2014, a DCM&B programmer and I cotaught tranSMART during a hands-on lab session for a graduate level bioinformatics course, "Foundations in Bioinformatics and Systems Biology." During this one-and-a-half-hour session, we introduced the class to tranSMART and its interface via slides and hands-on exercises. The session was a success, and I was invited to teach it again in spring 2015.

This gave me the confidence to develop a workshop to teach tranSMART to a broader audience. My goals for this session were to introduce tranSMART to more members of the U-M community and to help new users feel more comfortable with the platform. I believe that hands-on training is beneficial as it gives attendees the opportunity to learn via action in addition to watching and listening to a presenter. Video tutorials and user manuals are important instructional resources, but offering a hands-on training session provided a synchronous training opportunity for the local community.

In July 2014, a student and I cotaught the first openly available U-M hands-on training session on tranSMART. Under my mentorship, we jointly decided what features to cover and developed the course presentation. The student developed the workshop handout with specific steps, using handouts I provided her with from previous workshops as a guide. I taught a portion of the class, which allowed my student to learn from my instruction style, and she taught a portion, giving her real-world instruction experience. We held a couple of practice sessions where I provided feedback on her instruction style and prepared her for potential questions. I also gave her advice based on my past experiences; for example, I recommended creating backup slides in case the tranSMART platform stalled at the time of training.

The one-hour "Introduction to tranSMART" session was held in the Library Learning Center, located on U-M's medical campus. We presented an overview of tranSMART and then guided attendees through three hands-on exercises, giving them a taste of tranSMART's capabilities. We provided a detailed handout to all attendees, walking them through the steps required to generate summary statistics, a standard heatmap (a graphic representation of data in a matrix format with informational color coding), and a box plot with analysis of variance (ANOVA). An evaluation form, developed by my student, was provided to class attendees at the end of the session. Although only three people filled out the evaluation, the feedback was useful. In addition to a couple of free text questions, statements were presented with a scale of one to four where one represented "strongly disagree" and four represented "strongly agree." Two people answered the question "I am more likely to use tranSMART after participating in this workshop," and both responses were positive with one ranking this statement as a three and one as a four. The statement "The exercises effectively taught me to use tranSMART's Dataset Explorer tool" received two ratings of four and one rating of three, proving the value of including hands-on exercises when teaching this translational research platform. Although the class size was small, feedback demonstrates the benefit of offering hands-on training sessions.

This session expanded the reach of the platform within U-M and gave my student valuable teaching experience. In addition, this was my first time teaching tranSMART in an open session, something that I hope to do more of in the future as use of the tranSMART platform increases. As the platform improves, I believe more researchers will recognize its value and be interested in learning to use it. Providing hands-on workshops introduce more potential users to this platform and will hopefully increase its adoption and further translational research at my institution. In addition to continuing to offer this introductory session, I would like to offer a more advanced session in the future that covers several more complex advanced analyses and the option to upload a gene list.

TOOL EVALUATION

When the tranSMART platform was introduced to the U-M community, several local research groups expressed an interest in exploring it further to determine if it would meet their research and data needs. A local tranSMART team, made up of a local member from the tranSMART Foundation, several programmers (from DCM&B and the Bioinformatics Core), and me, was established to help these researchers evaluate the platform.

One example is a prominent U-M nephrologist who is a member of the Nephrotic Syndrome Study Network (NEPTUNE, http://www.neptune-study.org/), a network of centers and organizations across twenty-two North American locations focused on nephrotic syndrome research. This researcher believed tranSMART might be valuable as a data-sharing platform for NEPTUNE. However, before bringing it forward to the rest of NEPTUNE, he wanted to assess the platform within his lab.

We began the assessment with a series of weekly meetings including the local tranSMART team and the nephrology lab. Small working groups were formed to look into specific topics, such as security, analysis capabilities, ease of use, and other criteria deemed important by the group. A local version of the platform was installed specifically for use by the nephrology lab. Members of the lab ran through several use case scenarios based on data already loaded into tranSMART and generated a list of questions and concerns. Using my documentation, tranSMART knowledge, and access to tranSMART, I answered their questions as best as I could. In addition, I did a walk-through of the platform with one clinician, where she attempted to use the platform while I was present. I was able to answer some of her questions and observe how she wanted to use the platform and interact with its features. This was a valuable usability exercise as I gained insight on how a clinician or researcher would use the platform in a real-world scenario.

Initially, this research group had a number of serious concerns about using the platform. Many of these concerns stemmed from the difficulty they were having in loading their own data. However, working closely with the U-M tranSMART data-loading team, these issues were resolved. In addition, we held a series of remote conversations with other current tranSMART users to learn more about how they were using the platform. Participating in these meetings increased my knowledge of real-world use cases. At the end of the evaluation period, the lab voted to adopt the platform. Although not officially affiliated with the lab, I was a voting member with the research team. That I was invited to vote expressed the extent to which this group valued my opinion and my role in helping them evaluate the platform.

The research team recommended the platform to the rest of NEPTUNE, and it was adopted. Since the evaluation period ended, I have supplied training materials that have been updated by the research team with NEPTUNE-specific information. Two members of the U-M nephrology lab attended my "Introduction to tranSMART" training class to further familiarize themselves with the platform and to get answers to a series of questions. In addition, lab members periodically e-mail me with tranSMART-related questions; they clearly see me as a point of contact for questions regarding the use of the platform. Participating in the evaluation exercise with this lab has heightened my communication with many of its members and increased my knowledge of the application of tranSMART in a real-world setting.

Moving forward, I expect to continue interacting with this research group. Also, as other research groups on campus are considering tranSMART and will likely need to undergo a similar evaluation process, I expect to participate in these evaluations and provide training when needed. Being embedded into the evaluation process was extremely beneficial since it gave me a better understanding of the desires and needs of the researchers, in addition to strengthening my relationship with this specific translational research lab.

COMMUNITY

Ultimately, the success of tranSMART will rely heavily on the accomplishments of the tranSMART Foundation community, because this will lead to additional functionality, improved usability, and a wider range of publicly available data sets. From the beginning, the tranSMART Foundation was intended to provide a home for the tranSMART community. One important component for community building is to have a website where prospective members and users can get information about the foundation and the platform. Although a wiki existed for the tranSMART platform, there was no other website presence; this was an area of concern to the tranSMART leadership.

To address this need, the director of informatics infrastructure at DCM&B, who is now also the community manager and secretary of the tranSMART Foundation, asked me to assess the websites of similar open-source projects, such as Cytoscape, a network visualization tool, and Drupal, a content management system. I noted useful aspects of each site to inform the creation of the new tranSMART Foundation site. I also did a comparison of various development sites including Drupal and Google Sites to choose the most appropriate software for our needs. In late 2012, I drafted a proposal for a tranSMART website presence, highlighting the types of information I perceived would be valuable based on my research. In early 2013, I participated on a website team made up of U-M employees and tranSMART Foundation leadership. Although the actual coding and development of the website were outsourced, the team met regularly with the contractors to determine the best design for the website, appropriate content, and more. The goal was to create an initial site with basic information and a plan to increase the content over time. The team was charged with creating the website in less than six weeks, as it was going to be announced at the 2013 Bio-IT World Conference and Expo. This extremely short timeline presented a challenge, limiting the scope of the content initially included on the website.

As the community has grown, my role has changed to meet new, revised needs. Although I am no longer directly involved with the management of the website, I have provided feedback on certain pages, such as the Training and Tutorials page. I attend monthly community webinars via GoToMeeting and am a member of the Foundation's 3C Community Committee charged with promoting awareness, transparency, and communications around tranSMART, where I have been active in the User Guide and Training Working Group.[11] I have supplied the committee and the foundation with the video tutorials created at U-M, along with their scripts. In October 2014, I attended the tranSMART Foundation annual meeting. In addition to hearing a number of interesting talks on real-world successful uses of tranSMART, I networked with other tranSMART Foundation members and attended the foundation's 3C Community Committee meeting. Attending this meeting provided me with an opportunity to become more visible and for people to put a face with my name. I have continued to interact with multiple individuals whom I met at this meeting, further enriching my tranSMART experience and involvement.

CONCLUSIONS

This case study shows one way in which librarians can play a role in translational research. The effort in translational research portrayed in this chapter has been in support of a specific translational biomedical research platform, but the breadth of my role has spanned numerous areas of work related to the platform. Aside from information gathering, my tasks included website content management, instructional resource development, teaching, project management, mentorship, platform assessment, and committee participation. All of these endeavors have made me more visible to the local and global communities and have shown the value of having librarians involved in such projects.

The role of project manager and mentor serves an important and valuable way for librarians to get involved in translational research projects. Given the time commitment of my additional professional responsibilities, the nine tranSMART video tutorials we were able to produce would not have been created without the help of my students. My goal was to produce a quality deliverable while giving the students a unique educational experience. In return, they were given an opportunity to learn and hone new skills to help them in their future careers, and they walked away from this project with real-world experience that taught them about translational research, instruction, collaboration, and screen-capture software. At the end of the project, I had all the students write a short reflection about their experiences and provide me with feedback on the project and the mentorship they received. One of my students wrote: "Thanks to you, I've learned a lot about critically looking at material from the audience's perspective, contingency planning for workshops, understanding how attention to detail improves the overall instructional product, and balancing a project's progression when many different collaborators and stakeholders are involved." I feel that it is really important to give future librarians and information professionals the confidence, skills, and knowledge for them to feel empowered as collaborators in fields such as translational research.

The work discussed in this chapter was not without its own set of challenges. The tranSMART Foundation is a very complex organization since it consists of both public and private institutions in addition to these groups being geographically dispersed. Working with people across time zones, both in the United States and in Europe, created scheduling difficulties as there was only a small window of time that fell within everyone's regular work day. There were other communication challenges, such as the high level of effort required to know whom to contact for specific information. With so many groups and individuals working on the platform, it was hard to know when the newest release would be made available; this created obstacles to developing video tutorials and planning the hands-on training session. In addition, the platform itself had its own set of complications, such as a data-loading process that required many steps with a steep learning curve. Finally, while working with students created a more productive work environment, student turnover was high, which meant allotting time for each new student to learn the platform and get acquainted with their specific project. A certain number of challenges are unavoidable when working within a complex organization such as the tranSMART Foundation. It is therefore important to understand these challenges, make reasonable predictions about future challenges, and try to minimize their impact when possible.

There is no question that my biology background was beneficial for the work I discuss in this chapter. However, with patience and a commitment to spend the time necessary to learn and understand certain terminology and processes, a librarian with limited biology background could still be successful in this arena. One of the students I mentored lacked a background in biology, yet she developed outstanding video tutorials for using tranSMART. Despite her steeper learning curve, she produced numerous tutorials and cotaught a hands-on session, learning much of the science terminology simultaneously. In this situation, the strength of her information and instruction skills proved to be more critical than her biology knowledge. As a result, I implore interested librarians to pursue such activities even if they do not have a strong science background.

I plan to continue my involvement with the tranSMART platform and tranSMART Foundation. As a member of the 3C Community Committee, I hope to remain involved with the global community and its activities. I plan to continue providing instruction to the local community and expect that I will be involved in future assessments for local researchers considering adoption of the platform. As the community grows and its adoption increases within U-M, I expect that my role will continue to evolve as needed.

My engagement with the tranSMART community and platform further cemented my role as a partner in my institution's translational research activities. My ability to create instructional resources, disseminate valuable information, and communicate with researchers positioned me as an important member of the tranSMART and the U-M translational research communities. At the U-M, the chair of the DCM&B is a champion of the library; this has led to the inclusion of librarians as collaborators in many projects, including tranSMART. I believe that this relationship has been valuable and prosperous for all parties involved and could be a model for other institutions. Librarians have highly sought-after skills that prove to be an asset in a wide range of projects. All it takes is for one researcher to make this discovery and then the rest of the community will realize the benefits.

ACKNOWLEDGMENTS

I would like to thank Alex Ade, Kevin Smith, and Jean Song for their valuable feedback and support in the writing of this chapter. In addition, I would like to thank all the individuals whose interactions and collaborations with me are represented in this chapter.

NOTES

1. About the University of Michigan Medical School. http://medicine.umich.edu/med school/about. Accessed November 18, 2014.

2. Athey BD, Cavalcoli JD, Jagadish HV, et al. The NIH National Center for Integrative Biomedical Informatics (NCIBI). *J Am Med Inform Assoc.* 2012;19(2):166–70. doi:10.1136/amiajnl-2011-000552.

3. Department of Computational Medicine and Bioinformatics. About us. 2013. http://www.ccmb.med.umich.edu/about. Accessed January 14, 2015.

4. NLM Individual Fellowship for Informationist Training (F37) (PAR-06-509). 2006. http://grants.nih.gov/grants/guide/pa-files/PAR-06-509.html. Accessed January 14, 2015.

5. Athey BD, Braxenthaler M, Haas M, Guo Y. TranSMART: An open-source and community-driven informatics and data sharing platform for clinical and translational research. *AMIA Jt Summits Transl Sci Proc.* 2013:6–8. http://www.ncbi.nlm.nih.gov/pmc/articles/ PMC3814495.

6. TranSMART Foundation. About us. 2014. http://transmartfoundation.org/about-the -pta. Accessed November 19, 2014.

7. Scheufele E, Aronzon D, Coopersmith R, McDuffie MT, Kapoor M, Uhrich CA, Avitabile JE, Liu J, Housman D, Palchuk MB. TranSMART: An open source knowledge management and high content data analytics platform. *AMIA Jt Summits Transl Sci Proc.* 2014:96–101.

8. Canuel V, Rance B, Avillach P, Degoulet P, Burgun A. Translational research platforms integrating clinical and omics data: A review of publicly available solutions. *Brief Bioinform.* 2015;16(2):280–90. doi:10.1093/bib/bbu006.

9. Schumacher A, Rujan T, Hoefkens J. A collaborative approach to develop a multi-omics data analytics platform for translational research. *Appl Transl Genomics.* 2014;3(4):105– 8. doi:10.1016/j.atg.2014.09.010.

10. Creative Commons Attribution 3.0 United States. https://creativecommons.org/ licenses/by/3.0/us. Accessed January 15, 2015.

11. 3C Community Committee. 2014. http://transmartfoundation.org/community -committee. Accessed April 23, 2015.

4

Librarian Integration in a Working Group of the REDCap International Consortium

Jennifer A. Lyon, Fatima M. Mncube-Barnes, and Brenda L. Minor

ABSTRACT

With the rapid growth of translational science, novel opportunities have arisen for biomedical librarians to contribute in unique ways. Two librarians who actively supported research initiatives at their institutions using REDCap (Research Electronic Data Capture), a free globally utilized software system for collecting and storing research data, were invited to participate in the development of an electronic data-collection instrument library application (the Shared Data Instrument Library) housed in REDCap. The librarians assisted with the instrument curation process, governed by the REDCap Library Oversight Committee (REDLOC), by assuming primary investigative roles for determining copyright ownership and subsequently obtaining permission from copyright holders to adapt instruments into REDCap. Over time, the librarians' role expanded to include helping to assess validity and usage of the instruments and contributing expertise to committee discussions. Additionally, one librarian served as cochair of the committee in 2013–2014. Integration of biomedical librarians into the REDLOC demonstrates the value and applicability of librarianship skills in translational research support.

INTRODUCTION

The National Institutes of Health (NIH) launched the Clinical and Translational Science Award (CTSA) program in the early 2000s with the goal of coordinating research across disciplines, across institutions, and across the United States. We were involved in the work at their respective institutions: the collaboration of Vanderbilt University and Meharry Medical College received a Clinical and Translational Science Award in 2007, which was renewed in 2012, and the University of Florida received its award in 2008. As of 2015, sixty-two CTSAs have been awarded by the NIH. Vanderbilt serves as the lead institution for the nationwide consortium via an NIH Coordinating Center grant.

The strategic goals guiding the consortium are:

- Build national clinical and translational research capacity;
- Provide training and improve career development of clinical and translational scientists;
- Enhance consortium-wide collaborations;
- Improve the health of our communities and the nation; and
- Advance T1 translational research to move basic laboratory discoveries and knowledge into clinical testing.

Translational research "translates" laboratory discoveries into treatments and cures. Clinical research is the testing phase of those treatments and cures in the clinical setting among patients. The overall intent of the CTSA consortium is to accelerate and facilitate the translation of research from the bench to the bedside, and then to the community, through methods such as data sharing and development of information tools.

REDCAP AND THE REDCAP CONSORTIUM

To support translational research, in 2004 Vanderbilt University created REDCap, a secure web application designed to build and manage databases and online surveys for electronic data collection, under the leadership of Dr. Paul Harris.[1] Harris and his team purposed the software as a free, user-friendly data-capture platform for small- to medium-size clinical and translational research projects. Many years and many iterations later, the development team continues to update the software with applications and features that creative researchers and support staff have implemented in a variety of use cases.

The software supports multiple types of research as well as operational and institutional data projects. REDCap's key features include the ability to capture data in clinical research settings at a patient encounter level, the flexibility to allow multi-investigator or multisite collaboration, rapid and easy data-collection instrument design process, a curated library of validated data instruments, export in multiple formats for statistical program analysis, internal data checking and validation, user rights controls, and protection for patient health information.

Now used by more than 1,400 nonprofit, academic, and government institutions worldwide, REDCap software is provided free with an end-user license agreement to those who meet the qualifying criteria (for-profit use is not allowed) and who are able to support their own on-site installations both technically and administratively (there is no third-party involvement). This partnership of REDCap users and supporters, which includes most of the Clinical and Translational Science Awardee institutions, makes up the REDCap Consortium.[2]

The REDCap consortium aligned its objectives with the CTSA consortium goals, with separate functions, and operates in a self-sustaining mode. Vanderbilt provides the software and updates along with some support infrastructure and mechanisms, but the group primarily supports itself in day-to-day operations. REDCap administrators who maintain their institutional installations of REDCap have the opportunity to network on a dedicated listserv. User documentations developed by consortium members are posted to a shared wiki space as well. Weekly technical webinars are held to give administrators the opportunity to discuss and resolve issues with the development team and other attendees when the listserv is not feasible. Weekly all-hands meetings keep members updated on current and future software development as well as consortium activity. The REDCap consortium is an exceptional group of collaborators with a solid history of service to its members and to more than two hundred thousand end users worldwide. In addition, a REDCap conference (REDCapCon) is held annually to give members the opportunity to network, train, and learn more about how REDCap is supported at other institutions.

Besides these opportunities for participation, volunteers serve on several committees from the consortium and lead special projects. REDLOC is the largest of the six committees that are either active or in the initial development stages: regulatory (21 CFR Part 11, HIPAA) and software validation, field validation, plugins and hooks, FAQ (frequently asked questions), training materials, and REDLOC (REDCap Shared Data Library Oversight Committee).[3,4]

The REDLOC consists of two Vanderbilt coordinators (including author Brenda Minor, a project manager), two cochairs, and fourteen members (including two medical librarians, authors Fatima Barnes and Jennifer Lyon). This committee is responsible for vetting instruments for inclusion in REDCap's Shared Data Instrument Library (SDIL). The library is a repository of electronic data-collection instruments, already coded into REDCap format, that can easily be added to an existing REDCap project. These instruments include surveys, questionnaires, tests, scales, and other data-capture tools created, published, and validated (tested for dependability) for use by clinical and psychosocial researchers. Multiple domains are included such as quality of life (e.g., RAND SF-36), disability and physical function measurements (e.g., Barthel index), chronic disease self-management tools (e.g., PACIC), pain and morbidity scales (e.g., PADT™), and psychological and neurological indices. There are also large sets of data-collection forms and popular ontologies (e.g., PROMIS®, NCI, and BRFSS).

This instrument library saves researchers the time otherwise required to reformat existing instruments into REDCap and provides them with a curated set of validated, often-utilized instruments already prepared and copyright-checked for their use. The library fosters standardization and data sharing, enhancing cross-study and multisite collaboration. In addition to including curated instruments that have gone through a thorough approval and development process, the library contains non-curated instruments, also referred to as "bottom-up," that are shared by researchers after a low-level review process.

The curation process for validated instruments involves multiple steps. First, an instrument is recommended by a REDCap user through a survey submission process. The information is stored directly in a REDCap project (database) where processing workflow is tracked. Librarians are then notified of the new submission. A librarian will pick up the recommendation through a self-assigning step and begin the initial review process.

This initial review process includes verifying open-source (free) noncommercial availability of the instrument, obtaining author/copyright-owner permission for inclusion in the SDIL, checking the published literature for the overall level of use of an instrument and the presence of validation study(ies) supporting the specific instrument, and the feasibility of conversion to REDCap format. If the instrument appears to fit these criteria, it is then passed on to the entire REDLOC. The committee reviews the information gathered to determine if the instrument should continue on to the development stage. In development, the instrument is adapted into REDCap format by one committee member and tested by another. Thorough and prompt analysis by the librarian is extremely important in ensuring not only the quality of instruments that are included but also the efficiency of the committee's workflow processes.

In the early years of SDIL's development, Harris and his team explored the idea of bringing medical librarians into the instrument review process. They believed that medical librarians could bring an additional layer of expertise to REDLOC, improving the level of proficiency in areas such as document research, copyright and fair use issues, and proper citation. Librarians also have close connections with the research community, often participating directly in their studies, and have an understanding of user needs and the development of user-friendly interfaces. Additionally, librarians bring expertise in tracking hard-to-locate citations (for determining instrument authorship) and knowledge of literature searching and evaluation of studies (for use in determining levels of instrument use and quality of validation studies). At the consortium level, and in line with committee goals, librarians uphold broad concepts such as adherence to best practices for data collection and better promotion of training materials for end users. In the following sections, we librarians discuss our experiences as part of REDLOC.

THE LIBRARIANS

Fatima Barnes, Meharry Medical College

Founded in 1876 to teach former slaves to deliver health-care services to their communities, Meharry Medical College is the nation's largest private, historically black academic health sciences center with an enrollment of 802 students in the schools of medicine, dentistry, and graduate studies and research. The mission of the college is to improve the health and health care of minority and underserved communities and to conduct research that fosters the elimination of health disparities.

Meharry Medical College is noted for its leadership in diversifying the nation's health professions workforce, highly effective and innovative educational and training programs, enlightened health policy development, culturally sensitive, evidence-based health services, and preeminence in focused research that leads to the elimination of health disparities. In that vein, Meharry's CTSA leads the Community Engagement Research Core (CERC) focused on community health care and community physicians.

Officially, there are nine members of the Meharry component of the CTSA. I began supporting the CTSA when I joined Meharry as a bioinformatician in the Clinical Research Center six years ago. My job included creating various types of databases for research projects and clinical trials for clinicians and research nurses. When the REDCap tool was introduced at Meharry through the CTSA, I was trained as a trainer for the Meharry community. In collaboration with the research informatics personnel at Vanderbilt University, I ensured that guidelines and protocol of using REDCap to develop surveys and databases were being followed. This was an important part of end-user training that was accompanied by video tutorials that are constantly added and updated on the REDCap website. To date, I have created just over a hundred databases and surveys for a wide variety of clinical research projects.

When I learned about the REDCap Library Oversight Committee (REDLOC) in 2011 from the weekly Clinical Research Center's presentations conducted at Vanderbilt, I volunteered to assist with the primary investigative role for determining copyright ownership. This is the first step in a process to subsequently obtain permission from copyright holders before adapting instruments for REDCap and including them in the SDIL.

Jennifer Lyon, University of Florida

During my employment at Vanderbilt University Medical Center's Eskind Biomedical Library from 2000 to 2010, I worked with REDCap founder, Paul Harris, at the General Clinical Research Center prior to Vanderbilt receiving the CTSA. After he developed the REDCap software, I was one of its earliest users. I collaborated with Vanderbilt's nascent Institute for Clinical and Translational Research (VICTR) to use REDCap to collect data and database links on Single Nucleotide Polymorphisms (SNPs) identified in Vanderbilt's BioVU DNA Databank. When I left Vanderbilt to take a faculty librarian position at the University of Florida (UF), I continued to use and promote the REDCap software in association with UF's REDCap team and maintained contact with Harris through the CTSI (Clinical and Translational Sciences Institute) consortium and professional networking. In 2011 he informed me that the REDLOC within the REDCap consortium was in need of librarian members. I expressed interest, and he connected me with the REDLOC project manager, Brenda Minor. After a discussion with Minor regarding the duties involved, I accepted committee membership.

My initial responsibilities for the REDLOC focused on investigating copyright, ownership, and validation status for data instruments that had been requested by researchers at REDCap consortium member institutions to be added to the Shared Data Instrument Library (SDIL) of the consortium. These instruments included questionnaires, surveys, demographics forms, and other standardized data-collection forms useful for research purposes. I worked in collaboration with Barnes of Meharry Medical College and Minor to determine the feasibility of inclusion of a REDCap-formatted version of the instruments in the SDIL. Further, as my experience with the REDLOC grew, I accepted the responsibility of cochairing the committee for one year (2013–2014).

In November 2014, I moved from the University of Florida to Stony Brook University (SBU) in Long Island, New York. As SBU is not presently an active member of the REDCap consortium, I have taken a step back from committee involvement. It is my hope that SBU will develop and promote REDCap use, training, and support at some point in the future; even if it does not, I am considering continuing to provide assistance with the stage 1 investigation of copyright and instrument use permissions. Regardless, my more than three years of involvement with REDLOC taught me a great deal, and I believe that I have provided a valuable contribution to the team.

LIBRARIAN ROLES: OBTAINING PERMISSIONS AND VERIFYING INSTRUMENT VALIDATION

REDCap users are able to request the addition of specific instruments to the database. Upon receipt of an instrument request, Minor triages the request to one of the librarians, who examines the instrument, identifies the authors, searches for the initial publication of the instruments as well as articles relating to validation, and tries to find present ownership and copyright status. These steps are essential as REDLOC guidelines require all included instruments to be (a) validated in scholarly publications and (b) available for academic research use at no cost.

Searching for the author of the instrument usually begins with identifying the original developers of the instrument through a combination of web search and literature search. While some instruments are easily accessible with clear ownership, others require a lengthy process of backtracking citations and searching for current locations, positions, and contact information for authors. Once the original authors are identified and located, including contact information from universities or institutions, the initial contact is made via a standard e-mail to inform the author that his or her instrument has been suggested as a possible addition to SDIL. The e-mail also gives links to information on REDCap and REDLOC and requests permission to include the instrument in SDIL. To determine copyright information for a specific instrument, web search engines and literature databases are utilized. Some instruments are copyrighted to publishers; in these cases, permissions are challenging to pursue. Other instruments are made available online through foundations or institutes, both commercial and noncommercial; some of these provided web-based contact forms from which it is challenging to obtain responses. Requests are e-mailed to copyright holders at least twice before the REDLOC is notified.

To confirm the copyright and open-use status of every instrument investigated, Lyon or Barnes contacts the author, foundation, or institute distributing the instrument or another relevant authority who could grant permission to use. Once permission to use is granted, the information is sent to Minor who finalizes the permission agreements. In cases where use of an instrument requires significant fees; the authors, owner, or publisher are unresponsive after multiple contact attempts; or other complications are involved, the instrument is eliminated from consideration for inclusion in the SDIL. Acceptance or rejection status and details about the review process are recorded in the tracking database. If an instrument is rejected, the requestor is notified that the instrument cannot be included and of the reason for this decision.

Additionally, as part of the REDLOC, the librarians attended regular monthly online meetings of the group and participated in the committee votes to finalize acceptance of all proposed instruments after they had passed the initial permissions stage described above. All active committee members rated each instrument based on three major criteria: (1) could the instrument be converted to REDCap format without significant difficulty; (2) how solid was the validation of the instrument; and (3) how well used or well documented was the instrument in the published scientific literature. Validation was determined by searching the literature for the instrument-specific validation studies. In some cases, the presence of multiple peer-reviewed research studies using the instrument was considered satisfactory. Once the ratings had been collected, any instrument that required further consideration would be discussed at a monthly meeting until a final decision was made.

Participation in the committee also provided the opportunity to contribute to discussions and decisions on the structure, design, content, and management of the SDIL and its website. During the time that both librarians served as members, the committee developed a secondary instrument submission system that allowed REDCap users at consortium institutions to upload their own instruments to the library, constituting a separate set of "bottom-up" submissions. These are distinct from the "top-down" instruments that went through the ownership and validation investigations conducted by Barnes, Lyon, and Minor. As part of the team, Lyon was able to provide input on how those two sets of instruments would be accepted, processed, and made available to REDCap users.

Lyon also participated in other committee activities such as discussions of REDLOC internal procedures. For example, the committee extensively reviewed the issue of standardizing the coding methodology for the committee members who were tasked with converting the instruments into REDCap format. As a result, an instrument-coding development guide to standardize common procedures such as variable naming, numeric coding of responses, and scoring was created. The committee also discussed inclusion of standardized clinical trial reporting form sets (e.g., the Clinical Data Acquisition Standards Harmonization [CDASH] forms from the Clinical Data Interchange Standards Consortium [CDISC]) and other large sets of instruments from various sources. In one case, a research group from the University of Kansas offered multiple instruments already coded into REDCap format, which required the committee to make decisions regarding obtaining author and copyright permission, checking versions and validation, and reviewing the REDCap coding to meet established REDLOC standardization. Finally, for the one-year period of November 2013–November 2014, Lyon served as REDLOC cochair with Laurie Shackleford of Vanderbilt University. Her primary responsibility as chair was to lead the monthly meetings, keep the discussions focused, and ensure that plans for necessary actions were formed out of the debate.

CHALLENGES AND LESSONS LEARNED

There were a number of challenges faced during the process of investigating and confirming authorship and obtaining permission to adopt and use instruments in the REDCap SDIL. These included fundamental issues in backtracking through multiple citations and authors; difficulties in determining who controls copyright, ranging from authors to journal publishers and institutions; and lack of response of the copyright holders to committee inquiries. In at least one case, the primary author was deceased; luckily, one of the other REDLOC members was at the same institution and was able to work with the deceased author's colleagues to identify someone who could provide copyright permission. In other cases, while permission was obtained from the authors, it was discovered that it was also necessary to obtain permission from a publisher. Also, some authors were difficult to locate as they had retired, changed institutions, or changed careers.

Some authors were willing to share their instruments freely with researchers but wanted to be able to see exactly who is using their instrument and how it is being used. Usually, authors can do this through their own websites. Unfortunately, the committee can only track uses by institution and is unable to provide specifics about the studies, as the individual REDCap installations at each institution are not accessible centrally. Therefore only basic download statistics could be provided. A second problem arose in dealing with copyright holders who required financial compensation in exchange for sharing through the library, either from the REDCap consortium or from the individual users. At present, there is no funding source or support mechanism in place to handle those types of transactions.

Additional issues included difficulties obtaining permission from authors in foreign countries whose primary language is not English. Assistance in translating inquiry mails to French was provided by one of Barnes's colleagues at Meharry in a couple of cases. Additionally, there were requests for non-English versions of instruments available in multiple languages, Spanish versions in particular. This led to some serious discussion with the entire REDLOC group regarding the validation of translations of instruments that had been validated in English but not necessarily in the second or third language. This concern is still present and is being considered by the committee on a case-by-case basis.

Similarly, there were concerns about instruments that had multiple versions. In some cases, a different group of authors had taken an instrument created by another group and altered it in some way, often shortening it. This resulted in concerns regarding author permission and validation. Again, these issues have to be resolved in a case-by-case manner, which often required full committee discussion.

There has also been a great deal of discussion by the committee on how to deal with requests for clinical trial-reporting standards and large groups of instruments. As discussed above, some organizations and researcher groups offered big sets of related instruments or standardized forms. Of these, some were already converted to REDCap format and some required formatting. When the organization held copyright, obtaining permission was less of a concern, but this still raised issues of validation and use of standards. The REDLOC has considered whether to create a subgroup focused on standards or to recommend that the REDCap consortium create a separate committee to focus on this issue. As discussed above, there were situations in which a university research group would submit a miscellaneous set of forms they had adapted; this necessitated individualized copyright checking for each form, which was a time-consuming process.

Finally, there were areas in which the librarians and the committee discovered a need to streamline the process or improve record keeping. In particular, the initial assignments of instruments, and tracking thereof, to the librarians for evaluation were originally done by Minor in a somewhat haphazard manner. There were no specifics for issues such as how long the wait periods for author/copyright-owner responses would be or how many contact attempts would be made. As the number of instruments increased and the need for more formalized tracking of the process became clear, a REDCap-based instrument assignment and tracking database was developed. Additionally, the decisions on when to "give up" on an instrument were slowly standardized, albeit with some variability for unusual cases (e.g., a deceased author). As with many of the committee operations, some forethought in standardizing procedures in advance, rather than when difficulties became apparent, would be beneficial—this was an important lesson learned.

OUTCOMES AND FUTURE PLANS

When the librarians came on board with the REDLOC in December 2010 and January 2011, respectively, the SDIL contained eighty instruments with a total of

383 downloads. As of June 8, 2015, there were 907 instruments (655 curated plus 252 user submitted) and more than fifteen thousand downloads.

Continuing forward, Minor and the librarians are working on developing a better reporting system, using a REDCap database to report instrument status, record data on each instrument, and track progress of the curation process from initial copyright approval to final inclusion in the SDIL. Barnes continues to work on identifying copyright and permissions for new instruments as they are requested. And Lyon is working on developing a collaborative relationship with the biomedical informatics group at her new institution in the hope of developing REDCap use and services there.

CONCLUSIONS AND RECOMMENDATIONS

The librarians were able to provide significant expertise and assistance to the REDLOC even beyond the primary processes of searching for and obtaining copyright permission to use published, validated instruments. These contributions include refining and standardizing workflow, improving database structure and the user interface, advising on methods of instrument validation, and even providing leadership and coordination.

For example, librarians were able to assume a positive leadership role in the decision-making process on allowing "bottom-up" submissions from authors that were not curated through the "top-down" librarian- and REDLOC-mediated copyright and validation process. Many REDCap users developed their own unique forms for their specific projects and wanted to share them with collaborators or other researchers. Both librarians made recommendations that were incorporated in the committee's final decision to offer a separate uploading process for these user-submitted instruments, including dealing with issues of validation, wording of disclaimers, and website interface design.

This experience demonstrates clearly that librarians should not be afraid of seizing new opportunities outside of their traditional roles. In today's information-rich world, librarians have highly valuable skill sets and experience that can be adapted to different situations, particularly within interdisciplinary committees and teams. It is vital to encourage and maintain relationships with colleagues and patrons in a variety of disciplines, to express willingness to assume new roles and responsibilities, and to step forward when such opportunities appear. Volunteering for projects of interest or where librarian skills can provide significant impact is an excellent method of demonstrating the value of librarians not just to your own institution but on a regional and national level as well.

In this case study, all members of the committee benefited from librarian involvement; the librarians and the information technology, database design, and content experts all gained from shared knowledge and experience. Each individual's contributions were valued and respected within the collaborative framework of the nationwide consortium-based work group. The REDLOC—including its librarian members—has succeeded in providing a vital and growing resource for the RED-Cap consortium's members. This project demonstrates clearly that librarian skills in citation tracking, copyright, open-access issues, database structure and searching, and user interfaces and training can be applied to nonbibliographic databases and alternative types of projects on a national scale to support CTSA initiatives.

NOTES

1. Harris, PA, Taylor R, Thielke R, Payne J, Gonzalez N, Conde JG. Research electronic data capture (REDCap): A metadata-driven methodology and workflow process for providing translational research informatics support. *J Biomed Inform.* 2009 Apr;42(2):377–81. http://www.sciencedirect.com/science/article/pii/S1532046408001226.

2. REDCap consortium. 2015. http://www.project-REDCap.org/. Accessed March 30, 2015.

3. Obeid JS, McGraw CA, Minor BL, Conde JG, Pawluk R, Lin M, Wang J, Banks SR, Hemphill SA, Taylor R, Harris PA. Procurement of shared data instruments for Research Electronic Data Capture (REDCap). *J Biomed Inform.* 2013 Apr;46(20):259–65. http://www.sciencedirect.com/science/article/pii/S1532046412001608.

4. Balise R, Banks S, Barnes F, Bosler T, Carlin L, Chamorro C, Fernandez M, Geller R, Gutman D, Lee J, Li A, Lyon JA, Minor BL, Oppenheimer S, Sanchez L, Shackleford L, Xue M. REDCap Shared Data Instrument Library (SDIL); REDCap Library Oversight Committee (REDLOC). Poster presentation at 2014 REDCapCon, Park City Marriott, Park City, Utah, September 23, 2014.

5

Tailoring Library Support for a Community Research Fellows Program

William Olmstadt, Mychal A. Voorhees, and Robert J. Engeszer

INTRODUCTION

Washington University is a private, medium-sized university in St. Louis, Missouri. Its School of Medicine is world renowned in a variety of fields, and its clinicians practice in the adjacent Barnes-Jewish Hospital and St. Louis Children's Hospital, as well as at some clinical sites in St. Louis County. Washington University has had a Clinical and Translational Science Award (CTSA) since 2007, and its CTSA was renewed in 2012. Similar to other CTSA recipients, Washington University centralized its CTSA activities in a distinct entity, the Institute of Clinical and Translational Sciences (ICTS).

Washington University's health sciences library, the Bernard Becker Medical Library, has been a leader among health sciences libraries in providing unique forms of library-based support to the ICTS. Reorganizations at the library in the last ten years have created dedicated library positions supporting the community health, consumer health, science support, and bioinformatics missions of the ICTS.

Many of the faculty scholars included in the Washington University ICTS were also the leaders of a pilot community research fellows program beginning in 2013 and repeated in 2014. This case study describes two library staff members' work with this program. We discuss our individual experiences and summarize lessons learned from both years of involvement.

PILOT YEAR: 2013 (WILLIAM OLMSTADT)

I describe the pilot year of the library's involvement in the community research fellows program. I'd like to emphasize at the outset that my only involvement during the pilot year was to provide library support for the cohort; I was not involved in the design of the community fellows program, the selection of the research fellows, or the outcomes of their final projects.

My involvement began in early 2013 when I was approached by Melody Goodman, PhD, MPH, about presenting library services to the community research fellows program. Goodman was leading the pilot program, and as the public health librarian at Washington University, I had already worked with some of her colleagues, though I did not know her personally. This fellowship was a newly funded ICTS venture taught in a relatively new space on campus during the summer of 2013.

The program was designed to introduce community members to the academic research process. Through a combination of lectures and coursework, the fellows gain a better understanding of the language and techniques used by researchers, the role that research plays in improving community health, and how community members and researchers can work together more effectively to advance mutually beneficial research goals.

The initial cohort was fairly large; at least forty-five community members were selected for the intensive, fifteen-week, nighttime fellowship experience. Fellows had to be at least eighteen years old, live or work in St. Louis, and have an interest in minority health, improving research literacy, or reducing public health disparities. Prospective fellows were chosen based on applications, resumes, and reference letters. Students who completed the pilot program had the chance to develop a proposal and apply for portions of a pool of funding designated for community research fellows projects. For additional reference, including information about the fellows' proposals, the fellowship application process, and related logistics, the Washington University fellowship is described in a recent article by Coats and colleagues[1] and was based on a program described and evaluated in Goodman et al.[2,3]

Because of my schedule and the scheduling of the class, offering library services to the fellows meant creating new resources in a relatively short time frame—about a month. To maximize the value of the library services, my first step was to learn what characteristics I could about the cohort of fellows. I learned from Goodman via e-mail that not all participants chosen for the pilot year had college education or formal education in research methods, although some did. Some of them did not have *recent* college educations, and their previous library experiences may have been in the era of card catalogs, typewriters, and manual index searching. They also may not have had writing-intensive education experiences. Some fellows worked, and some needed assistance with public transportation to participate in the course. I was able to ascertain that almost all the fellows had Internet access, either at home or elsewhere. This was helpful to know as security restrictions in place at Washington University meant that the fellows would not be able to access library facilities after hours. Therefore, resources chosen for the course needed to be accessible via the Internet as much as possible.

The faculty was aware of the difficulties that the diverse skill level could pose in instruction. To address this, Goodman asked the instructors for the pilot year to remember the varied backgrounds and skills of the cohort when designing their instructional sessions and also to think about ways to engage the fellows and inspire audience participation in the presentation.

Given the mixed nature of the cohort, including their diverse educational backgrounds and experiences, I planned to deliver library services in two different ways. First, I would use our LibGuides platform to create a stable reference resource for fellows that they could use throughout the course. Second, I would create and deliver an instructional session in the fellows' curriculum, highlighting free databases and information resources in the St. Louis community, presenting basic search skills and tips, and reinforcing how to make the best use of local public libraries.

To compile relevant materials for the LibGuide, I began by analyzing the content for each week of the course. Goodman provided all faculty members with a full course syllabus, which made it easy to identify relevant resources for each week, as well as to understand the context in which I'd be presenting. While the full course was fifteen weeks long, the final three weeks of the course were designated for fellows to meet with community leaders and develop their research proposals to submit for possible funding. Since there were forty-five fellows, it would have been difficult to create LibGuide information customized for each individual participant. Instead, I chose to focus on gathering resources relevant to the twelve weeks of didactic content. To provide an organizational structure for the resources, I broke the twelve weeks into tabs across the top of a LibGuide, creating each week as a top-level page. I dedicated the front page of the LibGuide to general information, including direct links to local libraries and websites defining basic library and research terminology. Then, using the syllabus as a guide, I worked through each week, looking up key websites and suggesting additional resources relevant to each faculty presentation. A screenshot of the pilot year guide is presented in figure 5.1.

My presentation was scheduled for May 2013, approximately a third of the way into the course. After reviewing the syllabus to understand the context in which my presentation would appear, I created a PowerPoint presentation mapped to the learning objectives for my session. My primary focus was on access to information, beginning with the resources available through the Becker Medical Library. As I knew that coming to Becker would not be an option for many fellows (for reasons I'll discuss later), I encouraged them to use their public libraries and spent a good deal of time discussing this option. I covered how to get a public library card and strategies to make optimal use of the excellent local library systems in St. Louis City and County, through both in-person visits and use of remote resources. I also offered some strategies for making the most of in-person visits, including searching the library's catalog ahead of time from a work or personal computer so that if they were going to a library to retrieve physical items, their time would be used well.

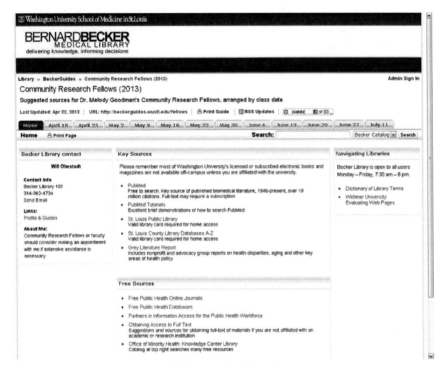

Figure 5.1.   Community research fellows LibGuide, pilot year 2013.

In terms of access to biomedical literature, I introduced the National Library of Medicine's PubMed (http://www.pubmed.gov/) as a free source for citations and abstracts for research or information about the fellows' possible topics of interest. I also covered PubMed Central (http://www.ncbi.nlm.nih.gov/pmc) for free full-text access to select papers. Finally, I encouraged the fellows to contact me with questions through the course and reinforced that I was available to work with them as they conducted research and investigated their topics of interest.

Goodman encouraged the faculty to inspire audience participation in the instructional sessions. Some faculty facilitated participation by breaking the fellows up into small groups for exercises, but I was not confident that this approach would work within the amount of time I had for my presentation (my session was scheduled with a longer presentation from another faculty member, and I had approximately an hour). To engage the audience and inspire participation among the fellows, I created two slides of multiple-choice trivia questions and dispersed these throughout my PowerPoint presentation. I used the American Library Association's most recent *State of America's Libraries* report to generate the questions, choosing things that would attract interest or get the audience's attention. Sample questions included the following: How many reference questions do librarians in the United States answer every year? How much money is spent on school library media and resources versus how much is spent on video games? The first person to guess—and shout out—the correct answer got a small giveaway. I purposely kept little free giveaways in my office for just such events: tote bags, pillboxes, pencils, and so forth. Using these general library questions as an icebreaker seemed to be a success—and the fellows were dismayed at how much is spent on video games in the United States.

Pilot-Year Challenges

There are always challenges in any program of this size, especially in its pilot year. The primary challenge I encountered was providing the fellows with convenient access to reliable information resources. During the pilot year, School of Medicine security restrictions prevented the fellows from obtaining official campus identification (ID) badges. This limited the fellows' access to the Becker Medical Library, whose doors are controlled by campus ID badges on weekends and after 6:00 p.m. on weeknights. Additionally, Becker Medical Library does not lend materials to the St. Louis public, which limited the fellows' access to print materials. Finally, fellows could not access Becker Medical Library's electronic resources off campus, as remote access is available to affiliates only. Having an ID badge would have made the fellows eligible for expanded library services, including borrowing privileges and badge-controlled access. However, given the short amount of time between finding out about the fellowship and the beginning of the course, I was not able to investigate and implement alternatives. I noted the difficulties this caused in the pilot and made a note to pursue this further for future cohorts.

In addition to the access restrictions, visiting the Becker Medical Library in person was not a convenient option for much of the cohort. Many of the fellows had to work during business hours (the only times they could enter the library without a campus ID), gasoline was expensive, and parking was difficult to find and rarely free. Due to these challenges, and given the fact that we could not give the fellows off-campus access to our electronic subscriptions, I chose to focus on freely available, high-quality information resources, such as PubMed and PubMed Central, rather than resources in our collection. I also emphasized free or low-cost alternatives to Becker Medical Library that might be closer to the fellows' residences, or more convenient than traveling to the central west end of St. Louis, including public libraries.

SECOND YEAR: 2014 (MYCHAL VOORHEES)

After William Olmstadt left Becker for a different position, the library was approached by the director of the community research fellows program to assist with the second-year cohort. As the person who filled Olmstadt's position, I assumed the responsibility. The second year of the program used the same structure as the pilot, and the experience and skills of the selected cohort were similar to the previous year's. The fellows came from diverse backgrounds and were selected for the program due to their high motivation to propose and learn about research that could directly improve the health of their community or population of interest. As with the pilot cohort, I was invited to present to the group and to deliver library services throughout the program.

To meet the information needs of the second-year cohort, I repurposed the original LibGuide. The organizational structure of the pilot year LibGuide was maintained, but I made several changes to tailor the guide to the unique needs of the new group of fellows. In particular, the second-year cohort was given a specific topic of focus throughout the fifteen-week program: obesity. While many of the original sources were still relevant, I updated the LibGuide to address the program focus, including additional resources specific to obesity-related community health, such as the Centers for Disease Control and Prevention's obesity and overweight resource web page (http://www.cdc.gov/obesity).

Olmstadt's PowerPoint presentation from the previous year was a helpful guide as I developed a similar presentation for the new cohort. I made use of the information he'd developed about using local public libraries, both in person and off-site, as well as other possible sources of help beyond the Becker Medical Library and specific online resources useful in community health and obesity. I also taught the fellows about methods and strategies for using Internet resources to facilitate their research. Like Olmstadt, I began with an introduction to PubMed (http://www.pubmed.gov/), promoting it as a source for citations with links to many free full-text articles the fellows could view at home, at work, or from a public computer. Due to the group's varied educational background, I walked them through use of PubMed, including how to do a simple search to find free full-text articles and how to use the PubMed tutorials for just-in-time assistance in the future.

In addition to PubMed, I demonstrated the use of Healthy People 2020 Structured Evidence Queries (http://phpartners.org/hp2020). These are preformulated queries that run targeted PubMed searches to retrieve evidence-based citations related to Healthy People 2020 objectives. I selected this resource both for ease of use and because one of the topic areas, "nutrition and weight status," was directly relevant to the cohort's focus on obesity. I felt these structured queries would be especially useful for those fellows who were not familiar with creating their own searches. I added these sources to the LibGuide so the fellows could access them throughout the course.

In an effort to encourage the fellows to participate and engage them throughout my one-hour instructional session, I also used a method similar to the trivia questions described. This group was very engaged and self-motivated; to capitalize on this, I encouraged questions and comments throughout the presentation, rather than taking all questions at the end of the session. I felt this open forum worked very well in this setting.

Second-Year Challenges

Unfortunately, in terms of library services, community fellows in the second year of the program faced many of the same access challenges as the pilot cohort. In particular, the Becker Medical Library was still unable to grant fellows badged library access, which would have made them eligible for expanded library services, including borrowing materials and after-hours access. For this reason, heavy emphasis was placed on alternative resources outside of the Becker Medical Library such as public libraries, other public academic libraries, and freely available online sources. Future programs should look at how this particular challenge might be overcome to provide fellows with an even richer research experience.

LESSONS LEARNED

There are always challenges to be expected when inviting the public onto college campuses. Below are the key learnings from both years of library support for the community research fellows:

- Start early, and be flexible with library policies. It may be necessary for health sciences libraries to adjust their policies (at least temporarily) to support translational research efforts that involve the community, including granting affiliate status for both on-site and remote access to program participants. If your institution is making this kind of fellowship a priority, it may be necessary to develop a mechanism for granting limited access to participants in these kinds of programs to ensure they have adequate access to information resources.
- Develop relationships: If library access is tied to campus security policies, it may take good connections to authorize a group of temporary fellows. It may also take time, so try to be proactive and don't leave this until the last minute. Maintain a good relationship with campus security and police; this may help in the long run.
- Be helpful and give tips up front. Consider any possible barriers the participants may encounter when visiting your library and be aware of their relative lack of experience in an academic library. If you were a guest, unfamiliar with your library and its resources, how would you like to be treated? What kind of information would you find helpful? Common questions may include availability of parking, public computers, and scanners. Be sure to mention any charges early on (e.g., photocopying).
- Understand your audience. The participants in the community research fellows program represent a segment of the community that many academic medical librarians rarely encounter. Our cohorts reflected a wide range of educational backgrounds; many had limited experience with technology and information resources and were unfamiliar with the tools and resources used by academic researchers. However, they all shared a passion for improving the health of their

communities and were open to learning about information resources that were not easily accessible to the general public. This presented a challenge to academic librarians to adapt their instruction methods to meet the unique needs of this audience and deliver effective training and support to connect with the fellows' background and experiences.

OUTCOMES

Our courses and materials were useful to the fellows in both cohorts in achieving their research goals. Sample research topics from both years are summarized in table 5.1. In terms of our specific library services, the offers for personal consultations were valuable but perhaps underutilized: During the pilot year, four fellows visited Olmstadt for additional assistance; three wanted assistance after the May 2013 presentation, and one came to the library to visit him during weekday hours.

In contrast, the response to the LibGuide was astonishing. Within two weeks of making it live for the first cohort, it was the seventh-most popular LibGuide for Becker Medical Library. Other ICTS faculty members appreciated the LibGuide so much that they requested it remain available after the end of the program as a permanent reference resource for the fellows. During the second year of the program, the guide was updated to reflect the emphasis the coursemaster had chosen to place on obesity research. The guide was visited more than 330 times during the course of the program with the most popular pages being resource lists related to community health, research methods, obesity prevention, health disparities, and cultural competency.

Table 5.1.   Sample research topics from community research fellows

Pilot Year (2013)	*Second Year (2014)*
The mental health of incarcerated individuals	Fellows worked on three major projects during the second year:
Using large data sets, such as the BRFSS (Behavioral Risk Factor Surveillance System)	• Healthy Body/Healthy Spirit, a health-education program in collaboration with a predominantly African American church in North St. Louis • The New Face of Homelessness, a study to assess the health needs of homeless women aged 45–64 • Creation of a Patient Research Advisory Board (PRAB) to build a collaborative framework between researchers and community members that increases research knowledge, advocates for community health concerns, and addresses health disparities

THE FUTURE OF THE COMMUNITY
HEALTH RESEARCH FELLOWSHIP

At the time this case study was written, the long-term future of the community health research fellowship program in St. Louis was unknown. For the immediate future, a proposal was submitted for a third cohort in the St. Louis region and was approved. The third cohort will begin in 2015, and the focus of this cohort will be research literacy. In addition to the St. Louis cohort, Goodman reports the program is expanding to Mississippi.

From the library's perspective, participating in the community research fellows program was beneficial in multiple ways. First and foremost, the program provided an opportunity for the library to directly contribute to improving community health in a way that fit perfectly with the existing resources and expertise we had to offer. The faculty researchers leading the project also saw how the library could support their work in ways that went beyond traditional types of library service. In this case, providing education and support for a community-based participatory research project serves as a meaningful example of a role that medical libraries can play in the process of translational science.

NOTES

1. Coats JV, Stafford JD, Sanders Thompson V, Javois BJ, and Goodman MS. Increasing research literacy: The community research fellows training program. *J Empir Res Hum Res Ethics*. 2015;10(1):1–10.

2. Goodman MS, Dias JJ, Stafford JD. Increasing research literacy in minority communities: CARES fellows training program. *J Empir Res Hum Res Ethics*. 2010;5(4):33–41.

3. Goodman MS, Si X, Stafford JD, Obasohan A, Mchunguzi C. Quantitative assessment of participant knowledge and evaluation of participant satisfaction in the CARES training program. *Prog Community Health Partnersh*. 2012;6(3):361–68.

6

Partners in Research

Connecting with the Community

*Kate Saylor, Molly Dwyer-White, Celeste B. Choate,
and Dorene S. Markel*

The effectiveness of clinical research relies on good communication from all stake-holders, especially the community for which the intervention is being developed. As access to health information, both high quality and otherwise, becomes more readily accessible online, consumers are taking advantage of resources other than their health-care providers to help make medical decisions. This rapidly expanding online community for health information has created a valuable opportunity for clinical researchers to contribute to the conversation, engaging with the public in ways that were once challenging.

Additionally, building public participation in the clinical research process is key to maintaining relevancy to the communities it seeks to serve. This interaction provides benefits for both the general public, in learning about potential new treatments for conditions, and the clinical researchers to help inform their research, tailoring it to the appropriate community. By establishing more opportunities to exchange information, community members and researchers will mutually benefit.

Establishing communication channels between the community, health-care providers, and clinical researchers is the first step to overcoming obstacles in increasing participation in clinical research. Poor communication between these groups has created a general mistrust of clinical research, which has halted the potential development of effective treatments. The oft-repeated statement "I don't want to be a guinea pig" reflects public lack of trust in clinical researchers. Molly Dwyer-White and colleagues reported, "Without new and improved approaches, recruiting research volunteers will remain a significant challenge for clinical research teams, particularly as limited funding necessitates smaller budgets and shorter timelines to engage participants."[1]

To address these needs, the Michigan Institute for Clinical and Health Research (MICHR), the University of Michigan Taubman Health Sciences Library (THL), and the Ann Arbor District Library (AADL) combined their strengths in a project: Partners in Research (PIR). The overarching goals of Partners in Research were to establish a partnership among MICHR, THL, and AADL to increase public interest and trust in biomedical and behavioral clinical research; raise the level of literacy, awareness, and participation in clinical health research; and examine the conditions that are optimal for increasing health research literacy and willingness to engage in clinical research over the long term.

Our partnership triad collaborated on several projects. We first tried to determine if the addition of social features to the web-based, clinical-research recruitment site increased public interest in clinical research. We then organized community health research forums hosted at the Ann Arbor District Library to determine if information presented in a public setting was an effective strategy for increasing public clinical and health research literacy, increasing public trust in health research, and transforming community members into community research leaders. The focus of this chapter is to describe the community events that provided a communication channel between researchers and the general public, distributed reliable consumer health information, and collected feedback through surveys and focus groups to determine the effectiveness of these interventions.

The purpose of these events, called health research forums, was to provide the general public with evidence-based health information and increased awareness of the importance of clinical research. The health research forums provided a rare opportunity for community members to "put a face to clinical research" and allowed them to direct questions to researchers. The forums addressed a variety of health topics (e.g., obesity, Alzheimer's disease, and breast cancer) in the context of clinical research and raised awareness of the importance of participating in clinical research. Outcomes were measured through health research forum attendance, responses to surveys, focus-group data, and the number of views of recorded sessions made available on the Ann Arbor District Library's website, as well as tracking the increase in people signing up for research studies.

FORMING THE PARTNERSHIP

As we moved forward to jointly address the public demand for current quality health-research information, health sciences libraries, public libraries, and academic research institutions seemed to be natural allies in addressing the need to improve health literacy. The University of Michigan (U-M) boasts of one of the largest health-care complexes in the world and one of the most extensive university library systems in the country. U-M has more than eight hundred million dollars in research expenditures annually. The diversity of these research activities, from medical to social and cultural, is a major contributor of Michigan's capacity for growth and development—and a major contribution to the Ann Arbor community. The Michigan Institute for Clinical and Health Research houses the National Institutes of Health's (NIH) Clinical and Translational Science Award (CTSA) at U-M. MICHR creates partnerships among units across the university, the NIH, external industry partners, and the community for both research and education. A component of MICHR CTSA is a community engagement program, which links and unifies existing programs into a collaborative and interactive network, and provides infrastructure and support for areas that need development.

Dwyer-White was the manager for the community engagement program when she learned about a unique funding opportunity, the NIH Partners in Research grant. The request for applications (RFAs) called for proposals from academic/scientific institutions and community organizations to forge partnerships: (1) to study methods and strategies to engage and inform the public regarding health science in order to improve public understanding of the methods and benefits of publicly funded research, and (2) to increase scientists' understanding of and outreach to the public in their research efforts.

Dwyer-White shared the RFA across campus with groups that were known to be doing community-based research, including the MICHR Community Engagement Coordinating Council (CECC), a group that consisted of community-based partners and university faculty and staff. Though THL was not a CECC partner at that time, Dwyer-White sought out the THL director, Jane Blumenthal, in case she might be interested in the health-literacy component of the RFA. Blumenthal was interested in the collaboration and also suggested connecting with AADL. After meeting with the team from the public library, which included Celeste Choate, associate director of services, collections, and access, and their outreach and programming staff, it was clear that there was synergy between the need to increase the public's awareness of research and the need for researchers to garner feedback from the community.

Partnering with the Ann Arbor District Library was a logical next step. The AADL is a trusted community institution that serves the residents living within the boundaries of the Ann Arbor school district from five library locations. As one of the largest libraries in the state of Michigan, AADL is committed to the community it serves through public ownership of print collections, digital resources, and gathering spaces for the citizens of the library district; responsible and sustainable growth; and promotion of community partnerships. AADL has a fully staffed community relations and marketing department responsible for event planning and for marketing AADL events throughout the community. AADL also actively engages with individuals, nonprofits, faith-based organizations, businesses, and community groups to develop and promote partnerships, services, and programs with a particular focus on reaching out to, and improving access to, services for the underserved. By drawing from strong relationships and customer service already existing at AADL, and providing AADL and their patrons linkage and greater access to U-M resources, this project launched long-term partnerships based on trust and equality.

The Taubman Health Sciences Library (THL) at U-M was a natural collaborator with both organizations. THL is a participant in the CTSA with MICHR and leaders in information management for biomedical and clinical research at U-M. In addition, the THL is a designated outreach library in the National Network of Libraries of Medicine (NN/LM). As an outreach library, THL provides health information to the local community and collaborates with the University of Michigan Health System and other U-M units in their community outreach programs. In recent years, THL has been awarded subcontracts for outreach to people with disabilities and to the public health workforce. The combination of the THL's expertise in health-information resources and the AADL's roots in the community was a strong foundation for collaboration to improve the health of the local population through access to information and to increase knowledge of and participation in clinical research.

To help guide the interactions and to ensure that each group felt the partnership was fruitful, we adopted the well-established "Principles of Good Community-Campus Partnerships":

- Partners have agreed upon mission, values, goals, and measurable outcomes for the partnership. The relationship between partners is characterized by mutual trust, respect, genuineness, and commitment.
- The partnership builds upon identified strengths and assets but also addresses areas that need improvement.
- The partnership balances power among partners and enables resources among partners to be shared.
- There is clear, open, and accessible communication between partners, making it an ongoing priority to listen to each need, develop a common language, and validate/clarify the meaning of terms.
- Roles, norms, and processes for the partnership are established with the input and agreement of all partners.
- There is feedback to, among, and from all stakeholders in the partnership, with the goal of continuously improving the partnership and its outcomes.
- Partners share the credit for the partnership's accomplishments.[2]

HEALTH RESEARCH FORUMS

The Partners in Research planning team organized eleven health research forums hosted at AADL from 2009 to 2010 on a variety of health topics relevant to the local community. Speakers, both MICHR researchers and community health organization representatives, were selected based on health topics that would resonate with the general public. Many of the speakers were of local or national renown in their fields, which generated great interest and attendance in those particular forums as well as the forum series as a whole. A thirty-minute question-and-answer session followed each presentation. The 2009–2010 lineup of Partners in Research health research forum events follows:

- March 2009: Genetic Risks and Cancer
- June 2009: Medical Innovations
- July 2009: Overcoming Obesity
- August 2009: Understanding Alzheimer's
- October 2009: Hungry Planet, Healthy Schools
- February 2010: Women's Heart and Health
- March 2010: OCD across the Lifespan
- April 2010: Low Vision and Glaucoma
- May 2010: The Other Women's Cancers
- June 2010: Prevention and Treatment of Type 2 Diabetes
- August 2010: From Illness to Activist: Kris Carr, Author of "Crazy Sexy Cancer Tips"

All health research forums were recorded and are available online through the AADL's website (http://www.aadl.org/video/collection/10). Video recording proved to be quite valuable for our community members; many attendees stated that being able to rewatch the presentations at a later time would be helpful to them as they learned more about the various conditions. The videos are still viewed regularly and as of June 2015 had nearly fifteen thousand views.

Most of the events featured information tables to provide resources for attendees. As a designated outreach library for the National Network of Libraries of Medicine, THL attends a variety of health-related events in the community to share high-quality, freely available resources for health information. At each Partners in Research event, Kate Saylor provided health-information materials to support each topic, including annotated bibliographies with relevant websites that focused on the health research forum topics, with selected print materials available through the AADL's collection. She also provided live demos of consumer health resources such as MedlinePlus (https://www.nlm.nih.gov/medlineplus) and NIH senior health (http://nihseniorhealth.gov/) and distributed information about other health information resources available through the National Library of Medicine.

SOCIAL MEDIA INTEGRATION FOR PROMOTION AND INFORMATION DISSEMINATION

THL played a large role in promoting these events. As part of the outreach program Saylor established for THL, the University of Michigan Library (MLibrary) Healthy Communities, she developed a social media presence to help promote consumer health websites, local community event information, and local health resources. Facebook and Twitter proved to be the most useful tools for communicating with our intended audience of local community members, health professionals, and health organizations. Utilizing our social media accounts, Saylor promoted each Partners in Research event to the online communities following the THL accounts.

Starting in the several weeks leading up to the event, Saylor shared event information to help increase attendance. During each forum, she also live-tweeted facts, quotes, photos, and links from the speakers' presentations. For the first few events, we created customized Twitter hashtags based on the event topic but eventually realized it was easier for the Twitter community to use a standard hashtag for the series, #aadlhealth. Using the same hashtag for each event also allowed our Twitter followers to create a saved search.

Sharing the information through Twitter also provided an opportunity for community members who were unable to attend the events in person to send questions along to the researchers. During the Q&A portion of the event, Saylor would monitor the feed, share Twitter questions with the presenters, and post their answers back on Twitter, replying to the user who submitted the question. Over the course of the two-year project, many of our tweets also were retweeted.

OUTCOMES

Partners in Research demonstrated a successful community-based model to improve the communication of health research information and opportunities for participating in clinical research. Based on event attendance, online viewing of recording forums, and survey and focus group feedback, the health research forums were a success. The forums provided a valuable venue for community members and researchers to raise awareness of the needs of the public and of the research community.

Additionally, these forums enabled more community members to register for clinical studies. During the events, attendees were provided brochures with information on the university's website and links to U-M's clinical studies portal Engage (now UMClinicalStudies.org). Due to substantial outreach efforts, including participation in the health research forums, we saw an increase in the number of volunteers that registered to participate in clinical research.

Finally, successful models from this project were implemented into the curriculum in community-based participatory clinical research for trainees, faculty, community members, and staff. Additionally, MICHR continued to work with THL and AADL to incorporate their involvement into specific community engagement program educational initiatives beyond the role of the R03 grant. This project allowed a new link to be made among a major research institution, an academic library, and the public library—an incredibly successful and balanced triad.

PROGRAM EVALUATION

Surveys

Health research forum attendees were asked to complete an optional thirteen-question pre- and postsurvey to identify and measure the impact of the event on their knowledge of and attitudes regarding clinical research. The surveys helped the planning team assess the concerns of the community as well as the usefulness of the data collected by the AADL and the researchers. Of the 928 people who attended the health research forums, approximately half completed the surveys.

While some of the responses to the questions that measure attitudinal change were left blank, we were able to prove a change in knowledge. On a scale from one (low) to five (very high), participants increased, on average, one level when asked pre- and postsurvey about their knowledge of clinical health research. On a scale from one (inadequate) to five (very successful), the average response from participants was 4.7 for how they would rate the programs overall.

Dwyer-White and colleagues reported: "One key theme emerged. Participants, if they had an opportunity to tell researchers what they thought, stressed on comments such as 'To get input and include (real) people in the community' and 'one of the biggest needs with regard to health research is making it accessible and understandable to lay audiences.' In sum, after participating in a Health Research Forum, audiences were moved to feel that they and others need more information on the subject."[1]

Focus Groups

Focus groups were conducted after most of the health research forums, usually within ten days of the event, to discuss ideal ways to learn about clinical research and ways to improve other outreach programs for the researchers. Motivation to attend the events centered on a few common themes such as personal risk of the discussed condition and a desire to be more informed to help care for a loved one and to learn about new treatments. Dwyer-White and colleagues found that "despite the overarching fears and mistrust regarding research, there ran an overwhelming desire for people to participate in research studies coupled with a strong indication that they would like more awareness of opportunities to learn about current research and ways to participate: People would like to be involved."[1]

The Q&A portion of the events, scheduled during the last thirty minutes, proved very valuable for the attendees. Many respondents indicated that scheduling more time for this portion would have improved future sessions. They also appreciated the university sponsorship of the presentations because it was indicative of the quality of the content; the institution's credibility helped attendees feel as though they could trust that the information being presented was reputable. This feedback was key in determining future work in the community to improve clinical research literacy, trust in the research process, and awareness of the importance of participating in clinical research.

CHALLENGES

Project Challenges

Based on early survey feedback from attendees, we determined that there was a lack of understanding in the connection between the health information presented and the clinical research that supports it. Some of the selected speakers were able to communicate this effectively, while others simply focused on the health topic. To help make the connection between the health information presented and the significance of the clinical research, the team developed an informational slide that discussed the link between health and the clinical research studies taking place at U-M. This slide was projected on the screen while attendees waited for the start of the session. We also added a comment to the welcome message that helped to reinforce the connection.

Partnership Challenges

As with any academic or community partner, the communication and management of time and expectations is critical. This project was heavily reliant on staff-level project management from the academic side—MICHR in this case. This was largely possible because of the R03 grant from NIH, which allotted dedicated time from each organization involved. Additionally, MICHR leadership viewed the parent project, "Engaging the Community in Clinical Research," as a vital project that would demonstrate how infrastructure support for community and clinical research partnerships could be powerful tools in expanding local outreach and new community-university partnerships.

NEXT STEPS/FUTURE PLANS

Funding for this project covered costs associated with planning and promoting events and focus groups over a two-year period, starting with the first event, "Genetic Risks and Cancer," hosted in March 2009, through the final event, "From Illness to Activist: Kris Carr, Author of 'Crazy Sexy Cancer Tips,'" hosted in August 2010. All forums were recorded and continue to be viewed online, but no additional effort was planned for future work on this project. Each member of the planning team has shared results of the program in various discipline-specific communities through published articles, conference posters, and conference presentations with the hope that a similar set of partners will utilize this successful model and program series.

LESSONS LEARNED

We have several suggestions for continued successful projects of this nature. The triad of a research center, academic library, and public library seemed to be very effective. This allowed for the delivery of information on research, the connection to resources at the library not only on research opportunities and knowledge but also on health data and information, and hosting the health research forums in a trusted place—with a connection to world-renowned experts on the health topics important to the community (which the public library is in touch with and helped select). What was particularly strong in our case was the circle back—the questions that were raised in the audience about health topics and research specifically were routed back to the researchers, which improved outreach initiatives.

Each institution must be able to provide dedicated staff that can get the nitty-gritty work done. Projects benefit from a good balance between the higher-level, big-picture discussions between the principal investigators and the "on-the-ground" work of organizing and promoting the events.

Discussing and agreeing upon clear expectations and desired outcomes is crucial to the success of this or any project. Outlining the course and scope of our project at an early stage allowed us to continue with a big part of the model (helping identify speakers, promoting the events, and staffing tables at the events) once the funding was gone. It is also important to determine what takes place because of the individuals involved versus the institutional partnerships.

CONCLUSION

The Partners in Research program built a valuable communication channel for the public to learn more about and engage with health research information and for the researchers to get a better understanding of the community's information needs regarding clinical research. This model could be duplicated with little or no additional funding with partners that feature outreach as part of their missions. Most public libraries share a reputation for being a neutral and trusted community resource and could provide a venue for hosting similar events. As many funding agencies encourage or require public dissemination of clinical research results, we found that many of the researchers would have provided a presentation for the public without a monetary incentive. Thus, in addition to contributing to the public good, this partnership benefited a number of other people. Researchers appreciated the opportunity to discuss their research and to get a better understanding of the public's perception of their work and the general awareness of their research areas. Ultimately, this program established a solid partnership among the three organizations that generated many opportunities for collaboration.

ACKNOWLEDGMENTS

This project was supported by grants from National Institutes of Health grant number R03HD059620 and was also supported by the National Center for Advancing Translational Sciences of the National Institutes of Health under award number UL1TR000433.

NOTES

1. Dwyer-White M, Choate C, Markel DS. Increasing health research literacy through outreach and networking: Why translational research should matter to communities. *Health Educ J.* 2015;74(2):144–55.

2. Meyer D, Armstrong-Coben A, Batista M. How a community-based organization and an academic health center are creating an effective partnership for training and service. *Acad Med.* 2005;80(4):327–33.

7

Developing an Educational Role in a Clinical and Translational Science Institute

Diana Nelson Louden

I like working with researchers. I like learning what they're working on, I like teaching them tricks that they can use in their daily work, and I like providing information that helps them do their job well. Developing an educational role as a translational research librarian working with my university's Institute of Translational Health Sciences (ITHS) has given me a forum to support individual researchers, as well as an opportunity to contribute to group efforts in support of the broader research community.

CLINICAL AND TRANSLATIONAL RESEARCH AT THE UNIVERSITY OF WASHINGTON

The University of Washington (UW) Health Sciences Library (HSL) strives to meet information needs in education, research, and patient care. We support students, faculty, and staff in UW's six health sciences schools, UW medicine, clinical sites in a multistate network, and ITHS. Although all of the HSL liaison librarians work with researchers, my position was created to focus on information needs of health sciences researchers—whether they are affiliated with ITHS, my other liaison groups (primarily scientific departments within the School of Medicine), or our broader health sciences community. As the biomedical and translational sciences librarian, I am responsible for creating programming and services for the University of Washington's "biomedical and translational research community"—a very large and nebulous group.

UW is home to a wide range of biomedical research—from regulatory DNA mapping to cardiac regeneration, HIV prevention, and patient-centered informatics tools. It has also been consistently one of the top recipients of funding from the National Institutes of Health (NIH), remaining among the top five public universities in terms of funding amount since fiscal year 1992.[1] In terms of total grant and contract awards received in fiscal year 2014, the six UW health sciences schools brought in $893,944,500.[2]

The Institute of Translational Health Sciences exists to provide research support for an even larger audience. It has an academic home at the UW in Seattle, but it encompasses a broad network of universities, research institutes, hospitals, and primary-care clinics throughout Washington, Wyoming, Alaska, Montana, and Idaho (WWAMI, pronounced "whammy"). This is an area covering 27 percent of the land mass of the United States.[3] The geographic reach of ITHS—which formed in 2007 as a result of a Clinical and Translational Science Award (CTSA)—matches that of the WWAMI regional medical education program of UW (figure 7.1). The WWAMI program relies upon collaboration among multiple institutions in multiple states to meet medical education and patient-care needs, whereas ITHS facilitates collaboration among many of the same institutions to meet biomedical research needs. In fact, ITHS has worked with investigators at nearly two hundred institutions in the WWAMI region.[4] ITHS offers research support such as pilot funding, assistance in identifying research collaborators, clinical research coordinator services,

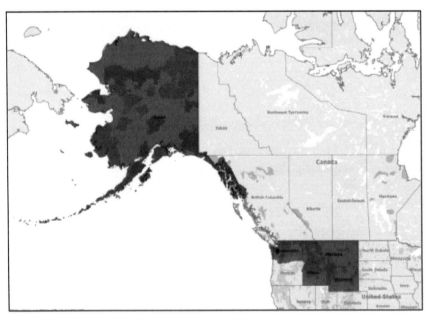

Figure 7.1.   WWAMI region. The designated reach of ITHS encompasses the same five-state region as the UW medical school.

and access to laboratory facilities and research centers. Experts within ITHS also consult on topics such as biostatistics and preclinical development.

Although I've worked with ITHS faculty and staff in several parts of the organization, my primary contributions in the past two years have been within their educational programs. These opportunities have arisen due to my regular participation in meetings of the Education Program Team (ED Team). Thanks to this existing infrastructure and receptive ITHS faculty and staff, I've had several opportunities to present seminars as part of structured learning and continuing-education programs. My relationship with ITHS education leadership also enabled me to develop a pilot project working with early-career researchers who have received KL2 career-development awards. (See the textbox on p. 80.) This aligns with ITHS's mission to provide the training and support needed by early-career researchers, as well as with HSL's mission of providing information resources and services in support of biomedical researchers. By identifying the information needs of KL2 scholars and determining effective means of educating and assisting them, not only do I contribute to the training of this particular group of translational researchers but also I learn how to better serve the broader population of early-career researchers throughout the UW health sciences community.

STARTING A NEW JOB AS A TRANSLATIONAL RESEARCH LIBRARIAN

Starting a new job as a translational research librarian was daunting. My job description left both the discovery of a niche and the implementation of appropriate services up to me. I knew that librarians at other institutions had established roles for themselves within their clinical and translational science (CTS) institutes, but I had no road map. In October 2012, I was a midcareer librarian accustomed to working with researchers in the biotechnology industry. I was new to academia, new to the UW HSL, and new to working in a grant-funded environment. I was in a newly created position envisioned and funded by the UW HSL, and no role or responsibilities had been identified for me within ITHS. I had been charged with developing a program of services in support of translational researchers within one year. This work was to be accomplished in addition to my work as a liaison to several departments in the School of Medicine, providing information support to UW biomedical researchers, working on projects with my colleagues, and learning to be an academic librarian. I would need to conduct outreach, assess information needs, identify opportunities, and provide useful information services to ITHS faculty and staff and the researchers they support. I was eager to get started.

I met with key people in ITHS, and I read constantly: about the CTSA program, about ITHS, and about what other librarians had done with CTS institutes. Extrapolating from the biotechnology research environment to the academic research environment, I generated a two-page list of ways I could work with ITHS staff members and the researchers they assisted. My director and I presented the list to members of the ITHS leadership in November 2012. The leadership was appreciative but did not seem immediately sure which of the suggested services could be useful to them or to ITHS-supported researchers. A small, but positive, outcome was that I was invited to attend a meeting of the ED Team in late January. And then I waited.

Having spent the first seventeen years of my career working as a biomedical and patent research librarian in a small pharmaceutical biotechnology company, I was accustomed to a fast-paced research environment, participating in ongoing projects, and nonstop research requests. By contrast, the next few months felt painfully slow. I met with a few more people. I was invited to a few meetings. I kept reading. My exact role was still unclear, both to the staff I met with and to me. A few people were under the impression that ITHS had funded my position. Others articulated needs of non-UW researchers and community groups that were outside my purview. I was anxious to *demonstrate* how I could contribute rather than *describe* how I could contribute.

Prior to attending my first ED Team meeting in January 2014, I learned more about the team and its role in ITHS. In 2012, ITHS consolidated their institutional structure into four major programs, one of which was education. This emphasis on education is in keeping with the goals of the CTSA program, which states that "a key component of the CTSA mission is the education and training of translational researchers."[5] ITHS's focus on education is also aligned with the recommendations of the Institute of Medicine's (IOM) 2013 report evaluating the CTSA program. One of IOM's seven recommendations was to "continue to emphasize innovative training, mentoring, and education to better prepare the next generation of researchers."[6]

The faculty and staff that are part of the ITHS ED Team offer both structured learning programs and continuing-education opportunities. Structured learning programs include a multiyear KL2 Mentored Clinical Research Scholar Program—a career-development award for postdoctoral scholars—and a TL1 Clinical Research Training Program for predoctoral trainees. Continuing-education programs include monthly seminars, grant-writing and REDCap workshops, a translational research "boot camp," and an online Self-Directed Learning Center.

At my first ED Team meeting, the group's faculty chair gave me a gift. She said I was welcome to attend meetings regularly without obligations so I could watch for opportunities to get involved. I was a sponge—learning about the grant-funded world, starting to understand the ITHS audience, and soaking up details about the educational programming the group offered. Within a month, the faculty member in charge of the ITHS career-development seminar series invited me to give a seminar on advanced PubMed searching for researchers. After a successful seminar in April, I started to feel that I was contributing to, as well as learning from, the ED Team.

DEVELOPING A PILOT PROJECT

While participating in ED Team meetings felt like a foot in the door, I was looking to make a more substantive contribution. In order to fulfill my goal of developing and implementing services in support of translational researchers, my supervisor encouraged me to develop a pilot project. Designing that project would let me define a discrete audience within my vast potential audience and tailor my services to suit that audience. A pilot project would also give me the opportunity to test ideas and assess their effectiveness. Another important benefit of developing a pilot project was that it allowed me, the librarian, to demonstrate how I could be useful rather than waiting for an invitation.

I also wanted to play to my strengths to increase my chances of making a valuable contribution to ITHS. I brought a scientific background, expertise as a biomedical and patent searcher, a genuine interest in the details and decision points of research projects, and many years of working directly with individual researchers and multidisciplinary project teams to ensure they had the information and skills they needed to conduct their research. With all of these things in mind, I took my supervisor's suggestion and tried to identify a group for a pilot project.

Based on my readings and research, I now understood that "translational research" was broadly viewed as research that incorporated knowledge from multiple realms in order to increase the speed at which research can improve health outcomes for patients and communities. With such a broad view of translational research and such a wide geographic region to cover, I realized how diverse and expansive the ITHS audience was. This confirmed my initial inclination: I didn't want my pilot project to be too far removed from individual researchers. It also posed a challenge: How could I decide what services to propose if I didn't know my chosen audience or their needs?

Although numerous assessment methods exist, the one I was most familiar with was an ethnographic approach: studying researchers by observing and talking with them in their natural environment. I identified three discrete groups of translational researchers supported by ITHS as possible target audiences, and I distilled my two-page list of ideas into a pilot-project proposal to be a dedicated librarian working with one or more of these groups. In the meantime, I kept attending monthly ED Team meetings and reaching out to the ITHS faculty and staff. At the April 2013 ED Team meeting—six months after I started at UW—I found my opportunity. The codirector of the KL2 Scholars program was sharing results from a survey of the scholars. When asked what they wanted to learn, the scholars had requested "advanced library training." He leaned over to look at me. I had received a second gift: the number one group on my pilot project list wanted a library seminar.

Over the summer I turned a seminar invitation into a plan for a nine-month pilot project. The KL2 program offered an existing infrastructure and a discrete group of self-identified clinical and translational researchers. The pilot project would give me the opportunity to ascertain the researchers' information needs, provide individualized training and research support, and solicit feedback on effectiveness. In addition to helping individual scholars, I also hoped to translate what I learned in order to more effectively support the broader translational research community.

THE KL2 MENTORED CLINICAL
RESEARCH SCHOLARS PROGRAM

The KL2 Mentored Clinical Research Scholars Program is funded through the NIH's National Center for Advancing Translational Sciences (NCATS) as part of the CTSA initiative. Although implementations of KL2 programs vary from institution to institution, each CTSA institute uses these awards to help individuals with doctoral degrees develop their research careers. The goal of the program is to provide mentoring, training, time, and funding to new researchers so they can become successful, independent investigators in clinical and translational research.

The ITHS KL2 scholars program offers multiyear awards to early-career investigators who are senior fellows or in their first faculty appointments (textbox 7.1). They seek applicants from a broad range of disciplines, including dentistry, medicine, naturopathy, nursing, pharmacy, public health, and social work. Three to five scholars join the program each year and remain in the program for up to five years; many also earn a concurrent master's degree in public health, biostatistics, epidemiology, or bioethics. The objective of the program is to provide enough mentoring and support that—by the end of the program—each scholar will be in a position to obtain at least one hundred thousand dollars in independent research funding as a principal investigator.

TEXTBOX 7.1
Who Are the Current ITHS KL2 Scholars?

- Recipients of NIH Mentored Clinical Research Scholar Awards funded through NCATS as part of the CTSA program
- Diverse group with a wide range of health sciences training, including orthodontics, psychiatry, emergency medicine, epidemiology, surgery, cardiology, social work, oncology, pharmacy, pediatrics, and global health
- Appointments at University of Washington, Seattle Children's Hospital, and Fred Hutchinson Cancer Research Center
- Four cohorts of three to five researchers per year
- Seventeen postdoctoral scholars as of June 2015

This multidisciplinary group participates in a structured educational program, including weekly seminars, throughout the academic year. Their interdisciplinary focus is strengthened through weekly "work-in-progress" sessions where scholars report on their research and solicit input from their peers. Learning from their peers and guest speakers, each scholar gains an appreciation for the goal of translational research: to promote the movement of knowledge throughout the phases of discovery, development, delivery, and outcomes research in order to accelerate improvements in population health. The scholars also develop the translational research mindset of including multiple parties in research assessment and priority setting. The translational research mindset is described in this way by ITHS authors Kelley and colleagues:

> Assessment and priority setting activities serve as a bridge, connecting stakeholders within and across the stages of translational research to ensure efficient handoffs and facilitate the larger goal of delivering on the promise of scientific discovery. With common understanding of the problem and goals, interdisciplinary teams can be more effective in making successful handoffs to assure discoveries reach development, delivery, and outcomes.[7]

The KL2 award is just one of the K awards (career-development awards) granted by the NIH, and the University of Washington is home to many recipients of NIH K awards. In an analysis of the number of new K awards per CTSA institution during the period of 2006–2013, the University of Washington CTSA was deemed one of the "top 10 performing" CTSA institutions.[8] As noted by Guerrero and colleagues, although other K awards are not tied to CTSA funding, the K08 (clinical investigator awards) and K23 (mentored, patient-oriented research, career-development awards) funding mechanisms are also "geared towards supporting the clinical and translational researchers." Even though recipients of these other K awards are not part of the ITHS structured educational program, they are still considered an important audience for ITHS resources and programming. They would be considered an important audience for library resources and research support services as well.

THE FIRST ACADEMIC YEAR: A NINE-MONTH PILOT PROJECT

As part of their program, the KL2 scholars participate in weekly seminars throughout the academic year. The program directors invited me to give two of those seminars during the 2013–2014 academic year—one in the fall and one in the spring—and they left the content of the seminars up to me. Not knowing what kind of "advanced library training" the scholars would find most useful, I asked the directors if I could survey the cohort. I used the survey to introduce myself as their librarian, ask how they identified and managed the information they needed, gauge their familiarity with and interest in various research tools, and solicit their feedback on what they wanted to learn.

I received responses from all seventeen scholars and used their input to inform the development of educational content and research support. Knowing their commonly used resources and top interests helped me determine what content to focus on and how to deliver it. Here are some examples:

- The scholars were most interested in learning about current awareness alerts and advanced PubMed searching.

- Grant-writing resources were the second-most popular topic, so I added grant-writing content to an existing web-based Biomedical Sciences Toolkit and publicized it.
- Nearly all of the scholars used a citation manager—EndNote being the most popular—so during the year I sent an e-mail to the group with tips on maintaining a single EndNote library by syncing desktop and web-based libraries.
- Few scholars were interested in medical genetics databases, so I discussed this one-on-one with interested individuals rather than introducing this topic in a seminar.

Not only were the faculty directors receptive to my involvement in the KL2 scholars program, but also the scholars were very engaged. The day of my first seminar, three individuals asked to meet with me. Throughout the year my outreach efforts continued to be well received. Each time I made a presentation or sent out an e-mail, I'd receive at least one response from someone who wanted to follow up with me.

For my second seminar presentation, I focused on relatively new tools for publishing and grant-related activities. I talked with the scholars about ORCID, SciENcv, complying with the NIH public access policy, searching databases for funding opportunities, and using the research networking tools SciVal Experts and DIRECT-2Experts. Guidance on complying with the NIH public access policy was especially well received. This was due, in part, to a collaboration with the ITHS education program specialist who had talked with me in advance about the scholars' experience with NIH public access policy compliance. Together, we decided to focus on advice for building compliance into the scholars' publishing workflow. I added instructions and background information to the KL2 library guide, and the program specialist embedded the guide into the course-management website.

I relied on the assistance of many people that first year, including my library colleagues and librarians from other institutions. The HSL liaison librarians helped me understand the various work environments within the UW health sciences, topics that would be of interest to researchers across the disciplines, and information resources used by researchers outside my liaison areas, such as orthodontics and social work. During that time a particularly helpful article by Holmes and colleagues was published that included a list of library support activities that would suit the education and career development functions of CTS institutes.[9]

Once I began the pilot project, conversations with individual scholars were particularly enlightening. The program specialist had provided me with background information on each of the scholars, but each time I met with someone I gained a better understanding of their individual interests and challenges. After having spent many years working with people whose full-time job was research, I was amazed at all of the nonresearch duties the scholars were juggling. Scholars retain their clinical, teaching, or mentoring responsibilities: those who are junior faculty may be teaching classes for the first time or mentoring graduate students; those who are clinicians spend a lot of time involved in patient care. Those who are earning concurrent degrees in public health are also consumed by learning biostatistics and conducting research for their theses in addition to their KL2-funded research.

Given the many professional demands on the scholars' time, I focused on practical information—tailored to their situation—that could be readily incorporated into their research practices. I made the best use of meeting time by preparing extensively before individual meetings and following up with additional assistance afterward. No matter what they asked for help with, I attempted to help. They were quick to fill me in on their challenges and to explain the value of the assistance I provided.

These seminars and consultations provided the context I needed to think about what might be most useful for both individuals and the group. In addition to thinking about what sorts of information-seeking and information-management skills the scholars would want to develop, I started to emphasize ways I could help them be more efficient. Through a combination of individual research support, instructional seminars, occasional e-mail messages, and web content, I solidified a place for myself within the KL2 program that matched my strengths to their information needs.

ASSESSMENT OF THE PILOT PROJECT

At the end of the nine-month pilot project, I again surveyed the seventeen scholars. This time I enlisted the help of a librarian colleague with assessment expertise to examine the goals of my survey and craft questions accordingly. I was most interested in the utility of the content I had provided, the effectiveness of my information delivery methods, and the value of one-on-one consultations. I was also curious to know whether the scholars had incorporated new research practices in their daily work and which library services were worth continuing. Finally, I wanted to present a list of fifteen possible topics and solicit input on what they'd like to learn about in the following year. Textbox 7.2 shows highlights of the post–pilot project survey responses.

These formal assessment results, as well as individual feedback from scholars and program directors, confirmed that the services provided as the KL2 scholars' librarian had been worthwhile. Specific feedback helped me know what content to focus on in the second year and where to invest my energy. I found the pilot project extremely rewarding and was eager to continue working within the KL2 scholar program. I shared these positive responses with the directors of the KL2 program and headed into year two.

TEXTBOX 7.2
Highlights of Post–Pilot Project Survey Responses

Incorporation of content into research practices:

- Two-thirds of respondents (6/9) reported that during 2013–2014 they learned effective search strategies for PubMed and other databases, created/modified a current awareness alert, and registered for an ORCID ID.
- Five respondents had made more effective use of a citation manager, and four respondents had set up a SciENcv profile.

Utility of content provided by librarian: The most helpful topic covered by the librarian in her 2013–2014 seminars and e-mail updates was "current awareness alerts." This was followed closely by SciENcv and PubMed searching.

Effectiveness of librarian's information delivery methods:

- Respondents indicated that the most effective means for the librarian to deliver information was via presentations in the KL2 seminar course.
- All respondents who had had one-on-one consultations with the librarian (5/9) rated the effectiveness of this means of delivering information "very valuable."

Feedback on future librarian services:

- 89 percent of respondents rated librarian availability for consultations as the most valuable service KL2 scholars should be offered, followed by 78 percent who rated the delivery of an annual presentation as part of the seminar course as the most valuable service.
- Based on the librarian support they received in the KL2 program, eight of nine respondents are likely to seek out librarian assistance, or to refer a colleague to a librarian, for research assistance in the future.

THE SECOND ACADEMIC YEAR

The major challenge of the second academic year was the nature of working with a multiyear program. Each scholar's KL2 award lasted four to five years, so at the start of my second academic year, there were a number of transitions: five researchers had completed the KL2 program, twelve scholars remained in the program, and five new scholars joined the program. My audience the second year, then, fell into two groups: continuing scholars and new scholars. Most of the continuing scholars had attended my two presentations in the first academic year and would be in the audience again for my seminar presentation in the second academic year. What content could I present that would be useful but wouldn't duplicate material I'd already presented? In terms of the new scholars, how could I ensure that they had opportunities to learn material I'd presented the previous year, as well as provide input about content that would be most useful for them?

Since the new scholars hadn't been part of the post–pilot project survey in June 2014, the UW assessment librarian helped me develop a survey of interests and research habits of the five new researchers. With the opportunity to work with a small cohort of researchers from the beginning to the end of their multiyear KL2 award, I wanted baseline information so I could track what tools and strategies they incorporated into their workflows and research practices over the four- to five-year period. To that end, I asked about their use of current awareness alerts, citation managers, advanced PubMed search features, and approaches to literature reviews; about whether they'd written a data-management plan for a grant application; and about their understanding of NIH public access policy compliance. I also solicited the new scholars' input on what librarian services would be most valuable to them and what topics they were interested in learning about. I used the same list of fifteen suggested topics that I had offered in the June 2014 survey of the first group of scholars.

Five scholars granted permission for me to use their anonymous answers within the UW community; four of the five new scholars granted permission to use their anonymous data in professional publications. Highlights of the September 2014 survey results from those four individuals are listed in figure 7.2. Although training interests were fairly similar between the continuing scholars and the new scholars, there were a few interesting differences. The most obvious differences between the two groups' interests were in current awareness alerts and research impact. All of the new scholars (4/4) wanted to learn about current awareness alerts, whereas only 11 percent (1/9) of the older cohorts of scholars wanted the librarian to cover this

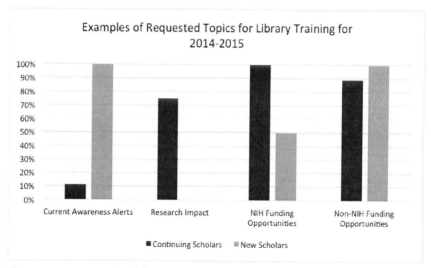

Figure 7.2. Noteworthy differences in selected training interests between continuing scholars and new scholars, 2014. (Responses represent nine continuing scholars and four new scholars.)

topic during the 2014–2015 academic year. Post–pilot project survey results had shown that current awareness alerts were the most popular topic covered during the 2013–2014 academic year, but clearly the continuing scholars wanted to move onto another topic. This was an essential tool that I'd need to address either individually or in a small group of new scholars.

Two-thirds of the continuing scholars were interested in "tools for describing research impact," whereas none of the new cohort was interested in this topic. A possible explanation for this difference is that members of the new cohort were initiating research projects and had not yet been faced with the task of describing the value of their research findings. Many of the continuing scholars, on the other hand, were applying for grants and needed to display their expertise and the worth of their past and proposed work. From a teacher's point of view, introducing the topic of research impact early in the researchers' careers seemed timely and important, so I made plans to address this topic in my seminar despite the survey results from the new cohort.

A third noteworthy difference between the two groups related to their interest in funding opportunities. While all of the continuing scholars (9/9) wanted to learn about finding NIH funding opportunities, only 50 percent (2/4) of the new scholars were interested in this topic. On the other hand, all of the new scholars (4/4) wanted to learn about finding non-NIH funding opportunities. The KL2 program director confirmed this trend by letting me know that several of the new scholars would be applying for non-NIH funds to continue their research. Although all of the scholars were supported by NIH funds through their KL2 award, I didn't want to focus exclusively on research tools for the NIH-funded environment.

With these survey results to guide me, I decided to present all new content for the second-year seminar. To address data-management needs, I invited the UW data services curriculum and communications librarian to present with me. She gave the scholars practical information on research data management, NIH data-management plans, and data sharing; I followed with tools for increasing and documenting research impact. I incorporated information about open-access publishing, citation analysis, networking, and altmetrics that would be applicable in many situations. I also introduced the Becker Medical Library Model for Assessment of Research Impact[10] and encouraged the scholars to track various manifestations of their research impact on an ongoing basis.

To give the new KL2 scholars a foundation similar to what I'd provided the scholars in the pilot year, I held a separate informal seminar with the five new scholars and also offered to meet with them individually. In the informal seminar, we talked about strategies for staying current with the literature, as well as NIH-related topics such as NIH public access policy compliance, My Bibliography, and SciENcv. The informal session was very successful in part because the researchers freely discussed their experiences, frustrations, and tips with their peers and me; it was an opportunity for everyone to contribute, ask questions, and learn from each other. I also had the benefit of a year's experience and could provide concrete examples of what the previous year's group of KL2 scholars had found useful. Due to the success of this approach, I decided to hold informal seminars and individual meetings with each new cohort of scholars.

SIGNIFICANT CHALLENGES OF DEVELOPING A ROLE AS A TRANSLATIONAL RESEARCH LIBRARIAN

My most significant challenge during the first year as a new translational research librarian was the ambiguity I had been warned about in the job posting. Not only was it unclear what my role and responsibilities should be, but also it was unclear who would decide what my role would be. At the same time, neither the ITHS nor the HSL environment remained static. I encountered staff turnover, changing directions, competing demands, problems, and opportunities. If clarity wasn't possible, at the very least I wanted to be able to discuss these challenges. Fortunately, my supervisor listened to me, helped clear up misunderstandings, advocated for me, served as a sounding board, and helped me navigate through unfamiliar environments. She helped me find ways to support the goals of ITHS, the goals of HSL, and my own career-development goals.

Although my role on the ITHS ED Team wasn't immediately clear, the faculty was familiar with the educational role of librarians and seemed comfortable with the ambiguity of my position. They approached me with teaching opportunities and asked me about information resources and assessment tools. Once my pilot project began, this gave me a substantive role, and the ED Team involvement gave my work a focus. From that position, it was easier to branch out to other parts of ITHS to offer assistance. Demonstrating ways I could be helpful was important to gaining acceptance.

Within the KL2 program itself, the primary challenges have related to the fact that the KL2 scholars are a multidisciplinary, heterogeneous group who are in different stages of their research careers and who may view themselves as primarily a clinician or instructor. As the scholars are learning from their peers, I'm using a combination of surveys, consultations, and classroom discussions to try to find areas of common interest across these varied disciplines. I'm not always successful. Because I work with a small group where I know each person by name, I'd prefer to be useful to each one. Still, I'm careful not to be too pushy. These are successful, busy people, and not all of them may see a need for what I'm offering. I keep the needs of the group in mind by presenting on topics of interest to a broad range of researchers. On the individual level, I focus my efforts on those people who seek me out.

The final significant challenge is dealing with the changing nature of the program itself. The challenges of supporting individuals in different phases of a multiyear program were described above. Leaders of the ITHS KL2 program also make changes in the weekly seminars based on feedback from scholars. Recently, there has been greater interest in peer-to-peer presentations than in outside speakers. The NCATS vision for the KL2 program is also changing. Funding for KL2 awards is shrinking, and KL2 programs will no longer necessarily be a part of all CTSAs. Starting with the current Funding Opportunity Announcement for Clinical and Translational Science Awards (PAR-15-304), NCATS may choose to fund a UL1 for a translational science institute without also funding a linked KL2 award.[11] Because of this shrinking funding, no new full-term KL2 awards will be made by ITHS in 2015. The KL2 program is continuing for the foreseeable future, however, and ITHS remains committed to training and mentoring investigators pursuing translational research. No matter how career-development awards change, it's likely that there will be some mechanism for me to provide librarian support to early-career investigators.

PROJECT OUTCOMES

The benefits of serving as the librarian for the KL2 scholars have been determined through multiple methods of assessment: formal and informal and documented and anecdotal. Because the pilot project was both rewarding to me and effective for the scholars, I plan to continue working within the KL2 program for the foreseeable future. As a librarian, I've benefited from working with the KL2 scholars in the following ways:

- Repeated interactions with a small group of people allow me to get to know individuals, see how they use information resources and tools as part of their work, and learn what they find both useful and challenging.
- What I'm learning and teaching as part of my work with the scholars can be repurposed for supporting other UW researchers.
- Establishing this role has led to other opportunities within the education team.

Based on the post–pilot project survey results, as described above, the KL2 scholars have also benefited. For example, most KL2 scholars had incorporated several things I had taught into their research practices, including current awareness alerts, new PubMed search techniques, and the NIH biosketch tool, SciENcv. In addition, all respondents who remembered and rated the usefulness of the 2013–2014 presentation and e-mail topics indicated that each topic was either "very helpful" or "somewhat helpful" (figure 7.3). They also gave valuable feedback on what support they wanted in the coming year. They requested additional library seminars and selected an average of eight topics (out of fifteen suggested topics) they wanted to learn about. Finally, they said that simply being available for individual assistance and consultations was the most valuable library service I could offer them.

In addition to conducting periodic surveys, I took notes on all individual consultations with KL2 scholars. For the period of October 2013–December 2014, eight of the original seventeen scholars and two of the five-person 2014 cohort have consulted with me individually, some multiple times. Although "occasional e-mail messages" was not a highly rated method of communicating according to the June 2014 survey, each time I sent an e-mail to the group, at least one person

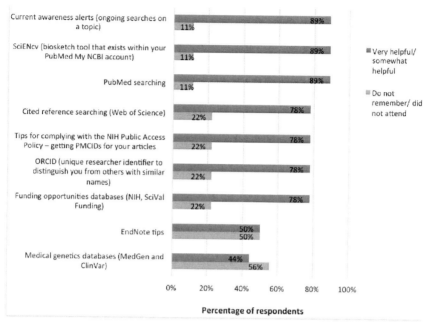

Figure 7.3. Survey responses in answer to the question "Which of the following topics covered in the librarian's seminars and e-mail updates were most helpful to you?" (Data based on nine respondents' answers at the end of the nine-month pilot project, June 2014.)

responded with questions and requests for assistance. Through individual consultations, I learned about their research projects, their phase in their research career, their work outside research, and how they used information and information-management tools. I've had opportunities to develop search strategies for systematic reviews, demonstrate the use of medical genetics databases to a clinician, brainstorm ideas for a research project for a master's thesis, provide tips on locating non-NIH funding opportunities, conduct searches on topics ranging from medical device information to survey instruments, and help several people make effective use of EndNote and current awareness alerts.

Although I've mentioned my focus on EndNote and current awareness alerts several times, it's worth emphasizing because effective use of these tools changes people's daily conduct of research, grant writing, and publishing. As one person told me, "You just saved me probably two hundred hours. Nobody shows you the basics; you just do what you need to get by." Gratitude for the basics was also echoed by another scholar who told me, "You've been more helpful than it probably feels like on your end—just to talk this through." Because of comments such as these, I was gratified but not surprised to learn that—based on the librarian support they received in the KL2 program—eight out of nine respondents were likely to seek out librarian assistance, or to refer a colleague to a librarian, for research assistance in the future. The scholars had been shown examples of how a librarian could assist them with their research activities, and when help was offered, they accepted. There were also several unanticipated benefits of serving as the KL2 scholars' librarian:

- Following my first survey of and presentation to the KL2 scholars, the directors of the yearlong TL1 training program for predoctoral students asked me to survey and present to their students. Now I'm involved in both structured learning programs offered by ITHS.
- Offering support to the KL2 scholars is an opportunity to also support the graduate students and postdoctoral fellows collaborating with the scholars. Although the scholars were being mentored by more senior researchers, they were also serving as mentors themselves; as a result, I was asked to teach literature-searching strategies to a graduate student and to help a postdoc with systematic review search strategies.
- The faculty directors of the KL2 program have given me autonomy, frequent encouragement, and timely feedback. They commented when they learned new things as part of my seminars and came to me with questions if they thought I could help. Most recently, one of the directors enlisted my assistance in assessing the effectiveness of our translational research training program.
- Finally, my work with the faculty and staff in the education team has made it easier to get involved in other aspects of ITHS's work. I've had opportunities to participate in projects and meetings, develop content for the ITHS website, and provide literature search support to ITHS faculty and staff embarking on projects or writing articles.

Becoming accepted as "the ITHS librarian" in this collegial network has provided me with opportunities to make meaningful contributions to the missions of ITHS and HSL.

LOOKING FORWARD

The ITHS KL2 scholars program continues to evolve. No full-term scholars joined the ITHS program in 2015 due to reduced funding for the KL2 program nationally. Also, according to recent feedback on the weekly KL2 seminars, the scholars have asked for more time devoted to discussions with their peers and fewer guest speakers. As a result, my role in the coming year may lean toward providing more individual support and web-based content.

While the KL2 program is contracting, ITHS has developed a separate faculty career-development program called Rising Stars. Beginning in 2015, this program will make two-year awards to promising early-stage investigators throughout the WWAMI region, thus extending the reach of ITHS's career-development offerings. Faculty members in the Rising Stars program will receive research funding, mentoring, peer-to-peer networking, and other services. Similar to the KL2 scholars program, the Rising Stars program aims to increase the number of early-stage investigators in the region who successfully obtain K- or R-series funding from the NIH for translational research. The Rising Stars program will provide another distinct group of researchers whom I can offer to support with individual research assistance, presentations, and web-based content.

Everything I learn while working with the KL2 scholars helps me provide more effective support to other biomedical researchers at UW. I learned from a clinician how he worked with genetics data. I learned from social work and public health researchers some of the challenges of interdisciplinary research. Information I learned about SciENcv, ORCID, and the NIH public access policy is now part of library guides available to the rest of the UW community. When I hear a scholar's honest recounting of the challenges of the new NIH biosketch requirements, I have insights that help me be more effective when I get biosketch questions from faculty in my other liaison groups. Even if the KL2 scholars program ended altogether, this small interdisciplinary group will have helped me in my efforts to provide useful support to the UW biomedical research community.

I'd also like to extend my support by adding content to the ITHS website to address typical information needs of researchers in the WWAMI region. The scholars have helped me understand I should focus on providing practical, time-saving, intelligence-increasing information. Now that I have a better understanding of the movement of knowledge through the various phases of translational research—from scientific discovery to outcomes research—I also want to provide information resources and guidance pertaining to each phase in order to help researchers who are accustomed to working within only one phase. For me, the KL2 scholars have been a microcosm for learning about the information needs of the translational research community.

RECOMMENDATIONS

As I began my new job, I faced the challenge of finding effective ways to provide library support to a vast community of clinical and translational researchers. Designing a pilot project gave me structure and focus, as well as an opportunity to explore what would be useful to a cross section of ITHS-supported researchers. I attribute the success of the pilot project to many factors, especially the receptiveness and interest of the individual people I worked with in the KL2 scholars program. For someone considering a similar project, I recommend: (1) utilizing existing infrastructure; (2) aligning the pilot project with the goals and strengths of the library, the CTS institute, and the librarian; (3) using what is learned in one setting to help researchers in other settings; and (4) incorporating assessment activities throughout the project to shape the content of instruction and services and to evaluate the usefulness of the project.

Consider Contributing to Existing Programs or Projects

When I was unsure how to get involved with my CTS institute, the existing infra-structure of the KL2 scholars program offered an opportunity to contribute to a high-priority program. I didn't need to seek out a suitable group of translational researchers because there was an existing group to work with. Weekly seminars offered a relatively easy way to engage with the scholars, and the small size of the group allowed me to be generous with my time and energy. I could offer both individual and group support and provide in-depth assistance on a wide range of projects without fear of overcom-mitting. I could also experiment with multiple methods of providing information before deciding which methods were most effective. The faculty directors supported my interest in assessment and facilitated my information gathering while helping me avoid contributing to the scholars' "survey fatigue." They also gave me autonomy to map out a useful role for myself within their successful multiyear program.

Align Your Services with Institutional and Professional Goals and Strengths

A new partnership between a library and a CTS institute (especially one where the librarian's position is not funded through the CTS award) should be aligned with the goals of both partners and should be consistent with the library's vision of service. In addition, although there are a multitude of ways librarians could work with a CTS institute, it's easier to demonstrate our value if we choose a project or service model that matches our individual strengths. Heading into an unfamiliar environment, I had a list of potential services so I would be ready to articulate how the library and I could help. With these possibilities in mind, I learned about ITHS's goals and core programs, and I watched for areas where I felt I could make a strong contribution. Rather than taking on the first project that was offered to me (managing NIH pub-lic access policy compliance), I instead created my own pilot project that built on the expertise and insights I had gained from working with biotechnology industry researchers. When I identified information needs outside my expertise (e.g., assist-ing KL2 scholars with data-management plans), I consulted with my colleagues and connected ITHS faculty and staff with other UW librarians.

Apply What You Learn from One Group to Assist Others

Our environments are always changing: people come and go, projects begin and end, and new opportunities emerge. As I worked with a small group of early-career researchers, I learned from our interactions and paid attention to what they found useful. I used this information to help the KL2 scholars, but I also got ideas for outreach, resources, and services for the rest of my liaison areas. For example, by monitoring changes in the NIH biosketch requirements and talking with a handful of KL2 scholars about SciENcv and biosketch writing, I could write a SciENcv Lib-Guide that was succinct and practical. The content was originally developed for the KL2 scholars but has since been publicized widely, resulting in workshop requests, troubleshooting questions, and lots of web-page hits from the UW community. Interacting with these seventeen individuals from multiple disciplines has helped me develop resources and services that are sensitive to the demands upon and interests of clinical and translational researchers generally. No matter how the CTS award system and KL2 program evolve, I'll be able to use what I've learned to assist other researchers—whether they are the ITHS-funded Rising Stars, recipients of other NIH career-development awards, or junior faculty in my liaison departments.

Make Judicious Use of Assessment

A pilot project lends itself to formal assessment activities. Knowing that I would want to evaluate the effectiveness of my instruction and research support at the end of the pilot project, I designed a survey to determine the scholars' initial familiarity with and use of tools such as ORCID, MeSH (medical subject headings), current awareness alerts, and citation managers. I also used the initial survey to elicit what the scholars meant when they said they were interested in "advanced library training." The initial survey supported my work in two ways: it gave me a baseline with which to compare future survey results, and it informed the content I delivered. I was able to deliver useful information the first time I met them because the scholars had already told me what they wanted to learn.

Throughout the nine-month pilot project I relied on informal assessment methods—from observing body language to documenting quotations from individual consultations. I was collecting information that would help me evaluate the effectiveness of the pilot project as a whole, but I was also learning from every e-mail and conversation. For example, when I saw that some researchers' projects bridged the health sciences and social sciences, I made a point to talk more about the value of databases such as Scopus rather than relying too heavily on PubMed. Informal assessment let me fine-tune the content I delivered and respond better to individual preferences and information needs.

For the formal assessment at the end of the pilot project in June 2014 (as described above), the assessment librarian and I wrote survey questions to determine whether my instruction and research support had been useful and what types of support the scholars found most effective. Since I wanted to continue working with the KL2 scholars beyond the end of the pilot project, I also asked what information content and types of librarian support would be most useful to them in the following academic year. In September 2014, I asked the same forward-looking questions of the new cohort of scholars joining the program. By considering the feedback from the first cohort of scholars along with the interests of the new cohort of scholars, I was able to decide what content to cover in my annual seminar (new content that matched the interests of most scholars) and what content to cover in a separate session of just the new scholars.

It was also extremely useful to ask the scholars which of eight potential services I should offer in the coming year. Survey responses indicated that they were most interested in annual seminars and having a librarian available for individual consultations. Seeing these clear preferences helped me focus my efforts primarily on these two mechanisms of support and not venture into less popular services such as developing web-based content.

With formal surveys bookending the project and informal assessment activities throughout the nine months, I was able to use assessment to shape the content of my instruction, evaluate the effectiveness of the services I offered, and tailor future methods of support to meet the needs and interests of the scholars.

CONCLUSION

Participating in the work of the ITHS ED Team has led to productive, rewarding work providing instruction and research support to multidisciplinary audiences. I've had the opportunity to learn firsthand about the ways ITHS develops and maintains support for researchers at all stages in their careers throughout the five-state WWAMI region. In my work with the KL2 scholars, I've also combined my favorite thing—working with individual researchers and helping them be more efficient and effective—with a project that has proved to be a great education in the challenges and successes of early-career investigators across the six UW health sciences schools.

At the time I planned my pilot project, all CTS institutes offered a KL2 program. Now NCATS has announced that they will not necessarily fund KL2 programs for each funded CTS institute. Still, as long as any of these CTS-sponsored predoctoral or postdoctoral structured career-development programs exist, they offer valuable opportunities for librarians' involvement with researchers, just as academic curricula offer opportunities for librarians' involvement with teaching faculty and students. Working with these talented early-career investigators puts librarians in the midst of fascinating research and intensive multidisciplinary training. While contributing to the success of CTS-supported researchers, librarians can also use these training programs as testing grounds for finding effective ways of contributing to the education and work of all of the researchers we support, wherever they are.

ACKNOWLEDGMENTS

The development of a translational research librarian role has depended on the insights, generosity, and support of many people. I thank my UW Libraries colleagues, the faculty and staff who work with ITHS, and the KL2 scholars.

NOTES

1. National Institutes of Health. NIH awards by location and organization. http://www.report.nih.gov/award/index.cfm. Accessed August 3, 2015.

2. University of Washington. *Annual report: Awards and expenditures related to research, training, fellowships and other sponsored programs, FY 2014.* Office of Sponsored Programs and Grant and Contact Accounting. 2015.

3. UW Medicine. WWAMI: Our regional training program. http://www.uwmedicine .org/education/md-program/admissions/why-uwsom. Accessed August 3, 2015.

4. Institute of Translational Health Sciences. Learn about ITHS. https://www.iths.org/ sites/www.iths.org/files/files/intranet/Learn-About-ITHS_031015.pdf. Accessed August 3, 2015.

5. Clinical and Translational Science Awards. Education and training. https://www.ct sacentral.org/consortium/education-and-training. Accessed August 3, 2015.

6. Leshner AI, Terry, Sharon F, Schultz, Andrea M, Liverman, Catharyn T, editors. *The CTSA Program at NIH: Opportunities for Advancing Clinical and Translational Research.* Washington, DC: National Academies Press; 2013.

7. Kelley M, Edwards K, Starks H, et al. Values in translation: How asking the right questions can move translational science toward greater health impact. *Clin Transl Sci.* 2012;5(6):445–51.

8. Guerrero LR, Nakazono T, Davidson PL. NIH career development awards in Clinical and Translational Science Award institutions: Distinguishing characteristics of top performing sites. *Clin Transl Sci.* 2014;7(6):470–75.

9. Holmes KL, Lyon JA, Johnson LM, Sarli CC, Tennant MR. Library-based clinical and translational research support. *J Med Libr Assoc.* 2013;101(4):326–35.

10. Sarli CC, Dubinsky EK, Holmes KL. Beyond citation analysis: A model for assessment of research impact. *J Med Libr Assoc.* 2010 Jan;98(1):17–23.

11. National Institutes of Health. Funding Award Announcement PAR-15-304: Clinical and Translational Science Award (U54). http://grants.nih.gov/grants/guide/pa-files/PAR-15 -304.html. Accessed August 3, 2015.

8

Expanding Research Networks

Judith E. Smith and Leena N. Lalwani

INTRODUCTION

Librarians and informationists at the University of Michigan (U-M), Ann Arbor, have embedded themselves in a variety of roles across campus to facilitate translational research. One way that we partner with campus clients is through the development and use of faculty-expertise tools. These tools hold the promise of helping users make connections to facilitate research and highlight expertise, which is especially important on a campus as large and complex as ours. U-M is a sprawling academic environment with nineteen schools and colleges, a research budget of $1.3 billion per year, and 128 graduate programs, one hundred of which are ranked in the top ten nationally.[1] As part of its research enterprise, U-M received its Clinical and Translational Science Award in 2007 from the National Institutes of Health (NIH) and developed the Michigan Institute for Clinical and Health Research (MICHR) to administer the award.[2] MICHR plays a large role on campus in enabling and enhancing clinical and translational research through funding assistance, education and mentoring programs, community engagement, research and management services, and other affiliated programs.

To partner with and support the diverse needs of researchers, students, and administration across campus, U-M has one of the largest academic research libraries in the world, the University of Michigan Library (U-M Library). As a library, our goals for involvement in translational research are not granularly defined. However, the overarching goals of leveraging our information expertise have shaped and propelled projects by librarians working individually and collaboratively to facilitate research and to be a partner in the research enterprise. This case study will focus on informationist and librarian involvement with faculty-expertise tools in primarily two libraries: the Taubman Health Sciences Library (THL—informationist, Judy Smith; translational research and data informationist, Marisa Conte) and the Art, Architecture, and Engineering Library (AAEL—engineering librarian, Leena Lalwani).

The process of translational research is "described as a 'translation continuum' because various resources and actions are involved in this progression of knowledge, which advances discoveries from the bench to the bedside."[3] Connecting researchers across disciplines is essential to move along this continuum, and tools such as Michigan Experts facilitate these connections and serve as key resources to forge new translational opportunities. Through profiling researchers beyond medical school faculty, as we describe below, researchers can identify others with complementary research interests. And, as librarians with a deep understanding of this tool and other types of faculty-expertise tools, we can partner with faculty to help make new connections. In this chapter, we present some examples of ways we have created opportunities to further translational research and discuss the challenges we faced and our future roles.

Both Lalwani and I have found that our involvement with faculty-expertise tools has not been confined to one particular project. It's more accurately described as a series of partnerships and projects that evolved over time and that are continuously changing to meet the evolving needs of our clients. Librarians can be described as a "campus conduit, helping researchers and administrators find resources and collaborators . . . a key way to serve the translational KFA (key function areas) whose goal is facilitating inter-institutional collaborations."[4] We embrace our roles as "conduits" in the broadest sense.

BACKGROUND ON FACULTY-EXPERTISE TOOLS

Faculty-expertise tools, also known as research networking systems, facilitate research in a number of ways. The tools are used to create profiles of faculty through their research outputs, which include awarded grants, publications, and patents. An additional benefit to the profiles is that they display subject expertise of faculty at both a high level (identifying general subject areas of knowledge) and a very granular one (specific topics in papers, patents, etc.) Taken together, these profiles highlight the scope and depth of research across disciplines in an easily accessible and trusted platform. Researchers can use that information to find collaborators; this creates more opportunities for both team science and interdisciplinary and translational research. Examples include commercial platforms such as Elsevier's SciVal Experts, ProQuest's COS Pivot, and Thomson Reuters's InCites, as well as open-source platforms such as VIVO, but a range of other tools exist.[5]

The content of each tool varies depending upon the sources used to feed the data; SciVal Experts ingests publications from Scopus, while COS Pivot pulls its data from ProQuest databases and from scraping the web. Some tools allow manual additions or edits by researchers or authorized administrators, including adding curriculum vitae or research interests. These tools often also afford universities the opportunity to brand the interface and reflect their unique institutional identities. For example, U-M originally licensed Collexis in 2009; this became SciVal Experts after Collexis was purchased by Elsevier in 2011, and our campus instance was subsequently branded as Michigan Experts (http://www.experts.umich.edu/).

As stated above, Michigan Experts receives its publications data from Scopus, and it also contains patents data, provided by the U-M Office of Technology Transfer, and grants data pulled from the U-M's eResearch Proposal Management (eRPM) system, a tool that tracks and processes sponsored projects. Update schedules vary based on the type of data; publications data are updated weekly, and the grants and patents data are updated quarterly. The tool offers three main ways of searching: by author name; by concept; and through a free text search that allows users to copy and paste text to be analyzed and matched to relevant researchers.

Presenting multiple types of data in a profile serves to help the user better understand the scope of the faculty members' work. In addition to the data mentioned above, a Michigan Experts profile provides information about a researcher's publication trend and coauthor networks and links to similar experts at U-M and other institutions. Another important component of the profile is the researcher's "fingerprint." This fingerprint displays the concepts that are most prevalent in a researcher's publications. The concepts are comprised of medical subject headings (MeSH) and terms from several other thesauri, including Compendex.

USAGE OF MICHIGAN EXPERTS ACROSS THE UNIVERSITY OF MICHIGAN

Before describing our specific roles, it may help to have a broad understanding of how Michigan Experts is used across campus. Below are examples of some of ways that Lalwani and I determined that Michigan Experts is utilized. We gleaned this information through our own experiences working with patrons and through interviews we conducted as part of writing this chapter. As U-M is a massive university, with thousands of faculty members, the uses below are intended to be a snapshot of usage across campus rather than a comprehensive accounting.

Publications Data

As at many other institutions, Michigan Experts is used widely by research administrators across campus to gather information about publication output as a way of measuring impact. Campus units from U-M's Cardiovascular Center to departments in the College of Engineering use data from Michigan Experts to create annual faculty activity reports, and various research institutes download and analyze data to see where their faculty members are publishing.

In addition to the Michigan Experts site, a local data warehouse stores a copy of publications, grants, and patents data from Michigan Experts. This warehouse is maintained by the Medical School Information Systems (MSIS), which updates the data pull monthly. MSIS's campus copy of this data provides the security of knowing that we have the data on-site. Additionally, while publications data can easily be downloaded from Michigan Experts, a local copy of the data allows clients to access and use data in ways that are not possible through front-end downloads. For example, ready-made, standard reports can be downloaded from a local software system, and ad hoc requests can be made to MSIS. Additionally, other faculty and administrators are using application program interface (API) to download the data. In some cases this data is used to update websites or publicize current lists of research outputs in specific areas.

Creating Connections

Michigan Experts is used in creative ways to make connections. The Institute for Healthcare Policy and Innovation (IHPI), an interdisciplinary health services research (HSR) group comprised of more than four hundred researchers, uses Michigan Experts to promote HSR to medical students as part of the Student Bio-medical Research Program (SBRP). This is a funded, mentored research program for first-year medical students, designed to encourage interest in basic, clinical, or translational research. IHPI participates in this program to introduce students to HSR opportunities and uses Michigan Experts to identify potential faculty mentors. Once a student provides areas of interest and a resume, an IHPI administrator reviews the Michigan Experts profiles of IHPI faculty to identify a faculty member who might be a good match.

Additionally, Michigan Experts data has been used to identify areas of faculty expertise and departmental needs when hiring faculty. Department administrators look at their own faculty members' strengths and existing collaborations, as well as upcoming areas of research, and analyze which areas could be strengthened by a new hire.

Analysis and Impact of Collaborations

In addition to creating connections, Michigan Experts data is often analyzed to better understand the value of these connections and collaborations. One current project tracks collaboration of researchers, staff members, and students over time. The project's overall goal is to see how moving to the U-M's North Campus Research Complex (NCRC) has impacted these researchers' collaborations from the time they moved into NCRC to the present. This is important for institutional planning, as a main goal of the NCRC is to facilitate interdisciplinary and translational research through co-location of academic research groups, as well as industry representatives.[6] This project is one way of measuring the NCRC's overall success in meeting this goal. In another example, Michigan Experts data was pulled from the data warehouse

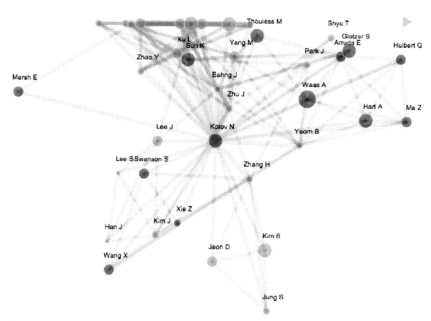

Figure 8.1. Sample collaboration visualization.

to analyze global publishing collaborations by the medical school. The faculty also uses the data to demonstrate existing partnerships or collaborations when applying for grants to highlight strengths in team science.

Figure 8.1 shows an example of a collaboration visualization that the front end of Michigan Experts can provide. The circles represent individual researchers, and the lines connecting them represent papers that they have published together. The size of each indicates the number of publications: a larger line = more collaborations; a larger circle = more publications.

Grant Opportunities

Michigan Experts enables a targeted distribution of announcements of funding opportunities or calls for research proposals. In the past, funding proposals were circulated to large numbers of faculty via e-mails or listservs. As is the case with many untargeted e-mails, the proposals were usually not relevant to most recipients, so they would go unread, in effect "training" faculty to ignore mass e-mail communications. With Michigan Experts, there can be a much more refined promotion. Administrators can search Michigan Experts by concepts in the funding opportunity, identify researchers with expertise in these areas, and push the funding opportunity notification to those researchers most likely to be interested. While issues still exist with the optimal mechanisms for distributing these targeted calls, the ability to quickly track down specific faculty members who may be interested in, or have the relevant expertise to capitalize on, an opportunity speeds up researchers' access to information about available funding. The U-M Medical School's Office of Research (UMMS OoR) also uses Michigan Experts to find reviewers for limited submission opportunities.

PHASE ONE OF LIBRARIAN INVOLVEMENT: COLLEXIS

The library's initial involvement with faculty-expertise tools began in 2009 through the work of our colleague Marisa Conte. At the time, Conte was embedded in MI-CHR, which funded a portion of her translational research informationist position. Conte played an important role in the development and implementation of Collexis, the first faculty-expertise tool used widely at U-M. In 2008, the UMMS chose Collexis as an ideal faculty-expertise platform for biomedical and life sciences due to its emphasis on data from PubMed publications and NIH grants. Collexis profiles based on these sources would give UMMS useful information to tell its "story" of strengths and identify areas for growth, as well the ability to identify strong collaborations and strengthen existing ones. Conte originally became involved when the key stakeholders and planners for Collexis, MSIS, and UMMS OoR reached out to the library to gain a better understanding of the controlled vocabulary that conceptually organized Collexis. She provided much-needed expertise on use of the medical subject headings (MeSH), including the value of major and minor headings and subheadings to refine faculty profiles.

As a result of these initial meetings, Conte became highly involved in product development. She participated in planning meetings with MSIS, UMMS leadership, and Collexis representatives as they began creating a prototype for approval by the UMMS dean. Conte helped the implementation team understand the data available in PubMed and defined various bibliometrics indicators, such as the h-index. Conte also assisted MSIS in translating ad hoc publications requests from users into queries that could generate usable data. Her knowledge of publication databases helped MSIS gain a deeper understanding of this type of data and facilitated their view of librarians as data stewards and partners.

Once U-M's Collexis instance went live, Conte was actively involved in UMMS-wide promotion and training. She conducted demonstrations at faculty meetings, departmental training sessions, and consultations with faculty and researchers. Additionally, she trained U-M's Collexis outreach teams on the type of questions and concerns the faculty would likely raise at product launch and demonstrations. Conte also conducted related work, such as data mining and producing publication reports. She used Collexis data to generate annual publications reports for schools, departments, and centers, including the Cardiovascular Center, College of Pharmacy, and Division of Hematology/Oncology.

Conte's initial presentations on MeSH to the development team led to a multi-year relationship with many significant outcomes, including ongoing participation with Collexis's development, drafting strategic reports for the UMMS dean, and the establishment of a solid relationship with MSIS to partner on other information-technology projects. Conte's work established the library as a true partner in the research enterprise vis-à-vis collaborative tools and expanded stakeholders' understanding of the range of expertise that librarians offer. This laid the groundwork for the library's continued involvement when Collexis was purchased by Elsevier in 2011 and was rebranded as Michigan Experts with an increased scope of research domain and integration of a broader content base.

PHASE TWO: EVOLUTION OF COLLEXIS TO MICHIGAN EXPERTS

When Collexis was purchased by Elsevier and rebranded as Michigan Experts, its focus expanded to include U-M researchers in the biomedical and life sciences, as well as engineering and other disciplines. The expansion of the platform was no small matter as this involved adding more than 1,200 new faculty profiles to the existing database. The interface also changed to more accurately reflect the complexity of the U-M environment. In the new instance, UMMS researchers could be searched by name or departmental affiliation, and users could also browse by certain institutes or centers, including the Biointerfaces Institute, Comprehensive Cancer Center, Frankel Cardiovascular Center, Kresge Hearing Research Institute, and Life Sciences Institute.

Elsevier's acquisition also had important ramifications for the content. The data source changed from PubMed citations and NIH grants to Scopus, a citation database owned by Elsevier. Integration of Scopus data allowed the platform to profile researchers in a broader range of disciplines. With a new data source and increased emphasis on facilitating interdisciplinary collaborations, profiles were built for faculty in the College of Engineering, College of Pharmacy, Institute for Healthcare Policy and Innovation, Institute for Research on Women and Gender, School of Dentistry, School of Kinesiology, School of Nursing, School of Public Health, Tauber Institute for Global Operations, and the Transportation Research Institute, as well as faculty from U-M Dearborn. Adding these disciplines benefited translational research because users of Michigan Experts could now identify collaborators with expertise in areas unknown to them to strengthen an interdisciplinary project. Moreover, researchers could identify and locate investigators in other disciplines that were interested in similar research. Since U-M is such a massive research institution, the potential for these interdisciplinary connections was strengthened.

To facilitate this expansion, the UMMS OoR created and led the governance group, consisting of representatives from each college or school represented in Michigan Experts. The group initially convened monthly and now meets at least quarterly. Conte did not participate heavily on the development of the new platform, though she continued to attend meetings about the product transition. She highlighted issues surrounding potential data-quality degradation as a consequence of moving to a platform with a new data source and facilitated contacts between MSIS and library personnel with expertise in product licensing, particularly for Elsevier's Scopus. To continue library involvement, I began to attend the governance-group meetings regularly, along with the University of Michigan Library's (MLibrary) core electronic resources librarian, who provided essential expertise on licensing issues. We worked together to identify other librarians with relevant expertise and invited them to attend specific meetings based on topic. For example, librarians spearheading the campus-wide rollout of ORCID (http://orcid.org/), a system to assign each researcher a unique and persistent digital identifier, presented on ORCID and its implications for units represented in Michigan Experts.

Attending the governance meetings allowed me to hear what was happening with the tool and to create further connections across disciplines. It became clear to me that a large part of our role with Michigan Experts was to function as an educator, a connector, and a translator. Since we work with so many clients across campus and varied disciplines and utilize many different information tools, our perspectives and experiences are broad. At a recent governance meeting, we brought up potential issues surrounding the pending conversion to the PURE platform, such as duplication of citations when importing publications data into PURE through other databases. We also made suggestions on more efficient ways to pull patents data from some of the existing databases. Overall, attendance at the meetings allowed other librarians and me to make new connections across campus, such as with the School of Dentistry, where I taught a Michigan Experts workshop.

In addition to making connections, attendance at the governance-group meetings allowed us to identify unmet needs and to partner in creating solutions. For example, the College of Engineering (CoE) expressed concerns that the Scopus data used to populate profiles in Michigan Experts did not provide adequate coverage of CoE faculty publications. At that point, Scopus's engineering data came from a bibliographic index called Compendex, and Michigan Experts was missing almost 30 percent of relevant data for electrical engineering and computer science. To address this gap, MLibrary's core electronic resources librarian and I contacted Lalwani, an engineering librarian. Lalwani quickly identified Engineering Village (EV), a publications database containing citations from both Compendex and INSPEC, as a possible supplemental resource. Lalwani analyzed EV's publication data, compared that to Scopus, and found that to make CoE profiles more robust, we would need to add these additional citations from INSPEC. Lalwani contacted INSPEC's creators, the Institution of Engineering Technology (IET) and obtained the necessary permissions to pull INSPEC data from EV to populate profiles in Michigan Experts. While this gave Elsevier the permission to pull INSPEC data, they did not immediately have the technical capability to pull that data for only U-M faculty at College of Engineering and to map the CoE faculty to the appropriate Michigan Experts profiles.

To this end, Lalwani identified and supervised a U-M School of Information (SI) master's student who wrote a script to clean up the data in a format that could be ingested into Michigan Experts. Additionally, she had to manually disambiguate common names (e.g., Wei Lu) to determine correct publication attribution. Once the data was cleaned up and in the right format, it was added to Michigan Experts. The increased completeness and accuracy of the data earned the confidence of CoE administration, which then determined they were ready to move forward with Michigan Experts. Lalwani's role was pivotal in ensuring that CoE faculty was fully represented in Michigan Experts and that CoE administration knew that their faculty publication data were accurately represented. Additionally, featuring accurate CoE data made it easier for potential collaborators in other disciplines to locate CoE faculty through Michigan Experts. CoE's resource planning and management expert mentioned during our interview with her that "librarians were lifesavers in getting INSPEC data into Michigan Experts."[7]

As MSIS began the process of implementing the new version of Michigan Experts, based on the new PURE platform, Lalwani has continued in this role. She conducted another analysis in October 2014 of Scopus's engineering-related data against EV's INSPEC data and found that the databases produced the same results for the engineering publications in 2013 and 2014 years. As Scopus now indexes recent publications from INSPEC, we decided it did not make sense to continue pull INSPEC data as it will result in duplicate citations.

In addition to serving as a resource for engineering data, Lalwani also provides expertise on patents data to governance stakeholders such as MSIS and the Office of Technology Transfer (OTT), the unit that had originally been responsible for providing patents data. OTT had been pulling this data manually, which is very time consuming and which caused significant delays in data availability. Lalwani has discussed the pros and cons of patent databases such as Derwent, Espacenet, Scopus, PubWest, and PubEast. Once Michigan Experts has completed its transition to the PURE platform, Lalwani and others will work on an automated process to pull patents data, which will facilitate more accurate records in a more timely fashion.

Participating in governance-group meetings has also facilitated another major role for librarians: education and promotion of Michigan Experts to different groups on campus. I was asked by governance representatives outside of my key liaison areas to provide workshops to their constituents on the benefits and use of Michigan Experts. To meet this need, I present one-hour workshops in which I provide live demonstrations of core features of Michigan Experts, emphasize its multidisciplinary nature, highlight the tool's collaborative purposes, and answer questions. Each workshop and specific search examples are geared toward the needs of the discipline, and I make an effort to include the library's subject liaisons when appropriate. For example, Lalwani and I cotaught workshops for CoE faculty and staff, and she was able to answer any engineering-specific questions.

Additional educational roles, while less formal, involve instruction and orientation to Michigan Experts through small-group or individual consultations. We provide many tailored information consultations to faculty, students, and staff across disciplines. Whether clients are new to campus or have been here for years, we include information about Michigan Experts and other research networking tools such as COS Pivot to our consultations whenever appropriate. We frame these tools as a building block for those seeking to make connections with researchers in similar or complementary disciplines. Even if our clients are not yet at the point of needing these connections, we work to increase their awareness so that the relevant research networking tools are on their radar. We also encourage students to explore research profiles and networking tools. We demonstrate how Michigan Experts and COS Pivot can be used to help students prepare for meetings with faculty members and identify potential mentors. We encourage both students and faculty members to consider contacting other campus researchers as another type of information gathering that can enhance their own research.

Another aspect of our work with Michigan Experts involves explaining the context and nuances of publication data. We receive many questions from clients across campus about the best ways to download publications data from Michigan Experts, the discipline coverage, data included, and export methods. Frequently discussed topics during consultations include publication coverage in the data provided by Scopus; the strengths and weaknesses of Scopus as a data source; and the different update frequencies of the public-facing front end of Michigan Experts (updated weekly, versus the U-M data warehouse, which is updated monthly). Additionally, we've worked with numerous users to help them understand their data-retrieval options. These consultations range from quick tutorials on how to download Michigan Experts data and import it into EndNote to recommending tools to help analyze the back-end data, such as NodeXL. Because these options can be overwhelming to users, we proactively try to create connections across campus to help solve problems.

Finally, the groundwork that Conte laid for our work with MSIS has formed the basis for an ongoing relationship. This relationship gives me a channel to pass user feedback back to MSIS who can implement changes to the local data warehouse or work with Elsevier developers to ensure Michigan Experts continues to meet user needs. For example, my work with units across campus demonstrated that clients needed to download accurate publication data at more frequent time intervals than what the front end of Michigan Experts can offer. I brought this to the attention of MSIS, who agreed this was essential to facilitate reporting. I worked closely with MSIS to define needs, clarify the data fields that were needed, and test the downloadable report generated from U-M's Michigan Experts data warehouse.

CHALLENGES AND LESSONS LEARNED

Our experiences working with Michigan Experts at all stages have highlighted the need for our unique skill set, including knowledge of information products and data organization and retrieval, to advance key areas of translational research. Using these skills is one way to begin partnering and building relationships that can result in larger projects. One significant lesson is that people often won't reach out to us, so we need to be present at stakeholder meetings to identify ways that we can partner and share our information expertise. For example, I learned about the College of Engineering's questions about publication coverage in Scopus at a governance meeting, not because they contacted me with a question. In other words, had I not attended governance-group meetings, I wouldn't have known about the need for better engineering data, and I wouldn't have involved Lalwani, who ultimately coordinated the ingest of this data into Michigan Experts.

One of the biggest benefits to working on Michigan Experts is the relationships and partnerships we've developed both through specific projects and through proactive relationship building. My work with the governance group has allowed me to build further projects with clients at NCRC, including working with the Biointerfaces Institute on best ways to retrieve publications data and to be more widely identified a "go-to" person for my liaison areas on questions related to publications data and metrics overall.

Lalwani's collaboration with engineering administration, mainly with the Office of the Associate Dean for Research, has helped her develop a closer relationship with the unit. This has, in turn, facilitated collaboration on many new projects, such as a data-management plan review services, and the introduction of successful workshops in publishing, copyright, grants, and data management. Engineering administration has also connected Lalwani with several departments that required assistance pulling data from U-M's data warehouse to generate faculty reports. Moreover, Lalwani forged a lasting connection with MSIS through her attendance at meetings, and she is now being included in other Michigan Experts–related projects, such as examining data integrity when publication data is ingested from different databases.

In terms of challenges, we are always looking for new ways to raise awareness of Michigan Experts. Although we provide instruction in formal and informal settings, it is difficult to maintain a high level of visibility of the tool and demonstrate its worth. Researchers who have been at the university for many years may not immediately acknowledge the value of Michigan Experts, as they may have preset beliefs about who is working on what across campus, or may be comfortable with the method they use to identify collaborators. Many researchers balk at the idea of a profile because they don't think it can adequately represent their expertise. Additionally, some researchers are not satisfied with their profile because it doesn't represent their current research interests and may, they believe, dissuade researchers from connecting with them.

As with any tool, our role in explaining the features and thinking of alternative ways to meet the needs is an ongoing challenge. We've recently encountered issues in how we teach the features and functionality of Michigan Experts. As we will be moving to a different platform with different layout and features in the very near future, a lot of the functionality will be changing. It's difficult to think of ways to engage users with the current platform, which may not meet their needs, while highlighting the upcoming new features. Additionally, there are always user complaints about some of the limitations of the current interface, including difficulties in searching by concept and then filtering results based on affiliation, or the inability to export data from the front end in formats other than .ris.

Finally, we often don't know or hear about the impact that Michigan Experts, or our work in refining and promoting it, has for our clients. Although we introduce them to Michigan Experts, we do not always hear the end result of how they used it, the outcomes, and what connections were made. Our clients are excited when they see Michigan Experts for the first time, but we don't have a deep understanding of how they use it, or what has been effective in our presentations so that we could subsequently tailor our efforts to facilitate collaboration.

NEXT STEPS FOR THE LIBRARIAN'S ROLE

This need for more information about the use and impact of Michigan Experts will inform our next steps. An immediate need is to help facilitate the transition of Michigan Experts to the PURE platform and to ensure that the end result is as usable and robust as possible. To succeed in this, we believe we need to develop a better understanding of how Michigan Experts is used across campus. We can work with key stakeholders, such as MSIS and OoR, to assess the use of the product across campus as a way of increasing its utility. This may also be a good point to find ways to assess our role in the process. For example, although we introduce many users to Michigan Experts, it is not always clear to us the direct impact this consultation and education has on creating interdisciplinary partnerships and the facilitation of trans-lational research. To further facilitate understanding of use, we could help organize users to share ways that they have used either Michigan Experts or the back-end data warehouse. And to increase use of Michigan Experts, we could create documenta-tion to share reported uses and outcomes, as well as nuances of the data and tips for queries and information retrieval. This documentation could take the form of online research guides or handouts in addition to being incorporated into educational ses-sions or presentations.

Finally, there will always be a new tool for identifying research expertise and building collaborations. As we learn of other tools that may be useful for facilitat-ing or analyzing collaborations, we can bring them to the attention of stakeholders and clients. For example, we are learning more about alternative metrics and will want to share these data and metrics with relevant users. We can also have an active role in partnering with MSIS and other stakeholders to decide the future directions of these expertise tools. The future of these tools may involve ingesting additional publication data, regularly or in an ad hoc fashion. Our skills in understanding the publication and licensing landscape can help facilitate potential content expansion. We can not only be a visible partner at the table to help coordinate interests and needs but also help on a granular level, such as working with MSIS to advise about data fields that may be most useful to clients as they consider pulling additional information from Scopus.

We envision that we will continue to play a highly visible role in education, specifically helping people across campus understand the ways that Michigan Experts can be used to facilitate collaboration. We also plan to expand our efforts to educate our librarian and informationist colleagues. Since our colleagues are in contact with many researchers across campus, educating them to use Michigan Experts will increase its reach and help promote the tool with the hopes of further facilitating collaborations.

We plan to continue our involvement with Michigan Experts because we feel we can play a key role in facilitating the interdisciplinary connections needed for translational research. We believe that our work with Michigan Experts has led to new projects and opportunities and that it has helped people across campus recognize the value of librarians as true partners, educators, and data stewards. Ultimately, we believe that research expertise or networking systems help to advance translational research, and we are strongly committed helping "translational research . . . venture out of its comfort zone and become more interdisciplinary."[8]

ACKNOWLEDGMENTS

Caleb Smith, Scott Dennis, Felix Kabo, Roohi Baveja, Linda Forsyth, Jason Wolfe, Laura Dickey, Mary Hill, Jennifer Hill, Millard Elder, Alec Gallimore, and Don Winsor.

NOTES

1. University of Michigan Office of Budget and Planning. Michigan Almanac. http://obp.umich.edu/michigan-almanac/. Accessed February 20, 2015.

2. Michigan Institute for Clinical and Health Research. MICHR overview. http://www.michr.umich.edu/about. Accessed February 20, 2015.

3. Drolet BC, Lorenzi NM. Translational research: Understanding the continuum from bench to bedside. *Transl Res.* 2011;157(1):1–5. doi:10.1016/j.trsl.2010.10.002.

4. Holmes KL, Lyon JA, Johnson LM, Sarli CC, Tennant MR. Library-based clinical and translational research support. *J Med Libr Assoc.* 2013;101(4):326–35. doi:10.3163/1536-5050.101.4.017.

5. *Wikipedia.* Comparison of research networking tools and research profiling systems. http://en.wikipedia.org/wiki/Comparison_of_research_networking_tools_and_research_profiling_systems. Accessed February 20, 2015.

6. North Campus Research Complex. About. http://ncrc.umich.edu/about. Accessed February 20, 2015.

7. Interview with Linda Forsyth. College of Engineering, Ann Arbor, MI.

8. Erler JT. Interdisciplinary research: Bold alliances aid translational work. *Nature.* 2015;517(7535):438. doi:10.1038/517438e.

9

Librarians' Roles in Translating Research Expertise through VIVO

Valrie I. Minson, Michele R. Tennant, and Hannah F. Norton

INTRODUCTION

The University of Florida (UF) is a large, public, land-grant institution, with more than four thousand faculty members and an enrollment of more than fifty thousand students. Based in Gainesville, the campus proper comprises sixteen colleges and includes an Academic Health Center (AHC). Six health-related colleges (dentistry, medicine, nursing, pharmacy, public health and health professions, and veterinary medicine), a hospital complex, and a veterinary hospital make up the AHC; it is "the country's only academic health center with six health-related colleges located on a single, contiguous campus."[1] The health enterprise of the university includes numerous clinics across the state, as well as a clinical campus in Jacksonville. The University of Florida also has a large agricultural presence, evidenced in Gainesville through the Institute for Food and Agricultural Sciences (IFAS), as well as numerous agricultural field stations throughout the state. In 2013, the university was conferred "preeminent status" by the Florida legislature, providing UF with at least seventy-five million dollars over the next five years to increase its research and educational presence.

The University of Florida's Health Science Center Library (HSCL) was founded in 1956 and is currently housed on three floors of the AHC's Communicore Building. Librarians at the University of Florida are faculty; when fully staffed, the HSCL comprises twelve librarians and one archivist, nineteen staff, and approximately thirteen full-time student assistants. The library serves the needs of Health Science Center (HSC) students, researchers, faculty, and administrators and is increasingly involved in the clinical enterprise through the provision of information services at the point of care (rounding and in the internal medicine clinic) and through a systematic review service. Additionally, the Borland Library houses a director/clinical librarian and a medical information services librarian at the urban campus in Jacksonville, along with two full-time staff members.

Through the liaison librarian program at the Gainesville campus, librarians are integrated into academic program instruction, collaborate with faculty on projects, and serve as "personal" librarians to the clients with whom they liaise. Liaisons are assigned to specific units (colleges/departments) or academic programs and develop subject-related workshops, perform in-depth information consultations, and provide collection development services for those units.

In 2009, the HSCL was integrated into the George A. Smathers Libraries, the library system to which all UF libraries (aside from the Legal Information Center) belong. One library in this same library system with particular relevance to the project presented in this case study is the Marston Science Library. Marston was founded in 1987 and serves the needs of agriculture, biological, chemical and physical sciences, engineering, and mathematics and statistics. Marston has eleven librarians (tenure or tenure track) and approximately eleven staff members.

UF's Clinical and Translational Science Institute (CTSI) was founded in 2008 and was funded by the National Institutes of Health (NIH) Clinical and Translational Science Award (CTSA) program in 2009. The goal of the CTSI is to "speed the translation of scientific discoveries into improved health by strengthening the university's ability to conduct clinical and translational research."[2] CTSI affiliates come from thirteen of UF's colleges with approximately 170 individuals paid at least in part by the institute and more than a thousand individuals utilizing the CTSI's services in a year. Organizationally, the CTSI runs through programs (units that deliver services to researchers) and governance groups, which provide guidance and a means for institute accountability. The CTSI provides numerous services in the support of research, including, but not limited to, regulatory and compliance, biostatistics, assistance with the data-capture system REDCap, quality assurance, reporting, ethics, and recruitment. Core facilities and resources such as the CTSI Biorepository, the UF Health Integrated Data Repository, the CTSI Human Imaging Core, and the Genotype Core are also available.

The CTSI also runs a number of educational activities for current students (MD-PhD, PhD with clinical and translational science interdisciplinary concentration, and master of science in clinical and translational science) and postgraduates (certificate in translational health science; the Training and Research Academy for Clinical and Translational Science), as well as a certificate program in basic coordinator training for research coordinators. The two-week summer course "Introduction to Clinical and Translational Research" (ICTR) provides researchers (including graduate students, fellows, and junior faculty) the opportunity to learn both the fundamentals of translational research and the resources available to them at the University of Florida. Although most centers and institutes affiliated with the AHC are served by the HSCL liaison assigned to the faculty member's department or college, UF's Clinical and Translational Science Institute is different. University leadership created and earmarked a new position, clinical research librarian, to work closely with the CTSI early in its existence. As such, the clinical research librarian provides targeted services to the CTSI, including instruction in and consultations for NIH public access policy compliance. This position also teaches in the MD-PhD program and in the two-week introductory clinical research course described above.

VIVO: CREATING A NATIONAL NETWORK OF SCIENTISTS

As early as 2004, Cornell's Albert R. Mann Library began development of a discovery tool called VIVO to support research collaborations, highlight the rich institutional research, and facilitate research funding connections within the life sciences. VIVO is a semantic web application containing profiles for researchers within an institution. VIVO has a shared ontology that describes people, organizations, activities, publications, events, interests, grants, and more. Data are added to a profile through dynamic ingest from authoritative local and external sources, including citation databases and grant or course information systems, or can be added manually (see table 9.1). In 2007, Cornell redesigned and enhanced VIVO using Resource Description Framework (RDF) and Web Ontology Language (OWL). This facilitated data sharing and data classification for machine-readable data.

UF's involvement with VIVO began in 2007 when two librarians at the Marston Science Library implemented a local version of VIVO called GatorScholar. The primary goals for this implementation were to serve as a tool to explore ongoing support for publication reporting to the United States Department of Agriculture (USDA) and to facilitate research collaborations across the entire institution. In 2009, the National Center for Research Resources (NCRR) of the NIH disseminated a call for grant proposals to "develop, enhance, or extend infrastructure for connecting people and resources to facilitate national discovery of individuals and of scientific resources by scientists and students to encourage interdisciplinary collaboration and scientific exchange."[3] While the contemporary UF and Cornell VIVO implementations were individual systems that served individual research communities, UF and Cornell were ideally positioned to apply for the award. In September 2009, a collaboration of Cornell, UF, Indiana University, Ponce School of Medicine, the Scripps Research Institute, Washington University in St. Louis School of Medicine, and Weill Cornell Medical College received $12.2 million in federal stimulus funding to create VIVO: National Network of Scientists. The vision was to use VIVO to promote the discovery of research and scholarship across disciplines within an institution with the overall goal of fostering team science.

Table 9.1.

Type of Data	Data Source	Method
Researcher data (name, dept., etc.)	Human resources (local)	Dynamic ingest
Publication information	Web of Science, PubMed, etc. (external)	Dynamic ingest with manual review
Grants	Division of Sponsored Programs (local)	Dynamic ingest
Presentations	Researcher, administrative staff	Manual entry
Courses	Course information system (local)	Dynamic ingest

Each VIVO profile (figure 9.1) highlights a researcher's unique accomplishments. VIVO further supports research discovery through data visualizations (figure 9.2) and the possibility of multi-institutional searches (figure 9.3).

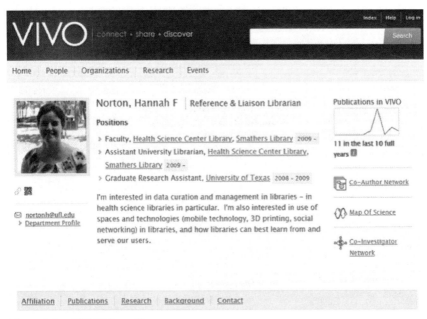

Figure 9.1.   UF VIVO profile.

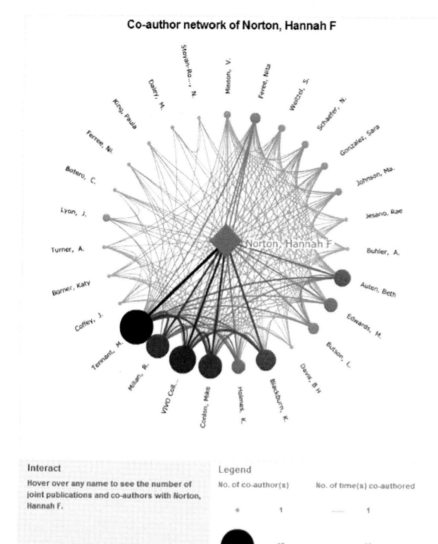

Figure 9.2.   Example of coauthorship network.

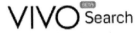

VIVO Search

Find research and expertise

norton | People | Q

People | Publications | Organizations | Activities | Health | Courses | Equipment

39 results

Norton,Barbara Jean
.. Assoc Prof of Physical Therapy Norton,Barbara Jean Norton,Barbara Jean Making decisions based on group designs and meta-analysis. Norton,Barbara ..
WashU in St. Louis School of Medicine

Norton, Mary Beth
Mary Donlon Alger Professor of American History
.. M Donlon Alger Prof of Amer Hist Norton, Mary Beth Norton, Mary Beth George Burroughs and the Girls from Casco: The Maine Roots of Salem Witchcraft ..
Cornell University

Norton,Hannah F
Reference & Liaison Librarian
.. Norton,Hannah F University of Texas at Austin Norton,Hannah F Norton,Hannah F VIVO: Are You Connected? Norton,Hannah F The Role of a National ..
University of Florida

Results by Institution

Cornell University | 25
University of Florida | 2
Weill Cornell Medical College | 4
Harvard University | 2
WashU in St. Louis School of Medicine | 3
Indiana University |
Ponce School of Medicine |
The Scripps Research Institute |

Results by Type

Figure 9.3.   Multi-institutional search.

VIVO AND CTS

VIVO has a natural relationship to clinical and translational science: both emphasize collaboration and the potential to bring together disparate groups with unique
resources and skills in order to further scientific discovery. In the NIH request for
application (RFA), the overall purpose of the project was described as "develop[ing],
enhanc[ing], or extend[ing] infrastructure for connecting people . . . to facilitate
national discovery of individuals . . . to encourage interdisciplinary collaboration
and scientific exchange."[3] This fits clearly within the purview of CTS, especially
given one of the specific objectives defined in the CTSA request for applications:
"Integrate translational and clinical science by fostering collaboration between
departments and schools of an institution and between institutions and industry."[4]
The CTSA program has helped develop institutional infrastructure for translational
research and collaboration and, at our institution and others, VIVO has become an
essential part of this infrastructure.

UF LIBRARIES' INITIAL INVOLVEMENT IN VIVO

The library's participation in the grant and resulting project provides an example of what can happen when library faculty and staff are (a) tapped into the needs of their users and (b) have an understanding of current library projects and priorities. The libraries' involvement was initiated after the director of the Health Science Center Library located the RFA and shared it with one of the authors (Tennant) of this case study who was already aware of the work that Marston Science librarians were doing with GatorScholar. She had previously introduced those librarians to CTSI leadership who had expressed a need and desire for a tool like GatorScholar. With this foundation already laid, it was a simple matter to bring the grant RFA to the GatorScholar librarians and the CTSI leadership less than a year after their initial meeting.

An interesting and unique aspect of the funding mechanism requirements was that at least seven institutions had to be involved in the project. Once UF librarians were aware of the RFA, we contacted the Cornell University team to determine whether that group would be willing to participate in a proposal; without their efforts a successful submission would be far less likely. Once Cornell was onboard, the two-institution team went about identifying additional partners, with the hope of developing a group more diverse than the two land-grant institutions. As such, the team sought a group of collaborators that included institutions both private and public, both research and academic, and both medical and broad based. Collaborators with particular skill sets were also important; for example, the data-visualization expertise available at Indiana University and the bioinformatics support offered by Washington University in St. Louis School of Medicine.

Roles and Project Life Cycle

Each participating institution set up a local installation of VIVO and created local implementation teams that served to feed knowledge to the national teams' collective efforts. VIVO teams at the national level included development, implementation, and marketing and outreach. Development work was accomplished at three institutions: Cornell led overall development work and the enhancement of the core application; University of Florida led development of the data "harvester" (a tool for pulling data from local and external data sources and attaching it to the appropriate VIVO profiles); and Indiana led the development of data visualizations and the ontology. Over the course of the project, as local data-mapping issues were identified, an ontology team was created to assist with local data mappings, identify local data that may be applicable across the multiple institutions, assist local stewards with accurately creating local extensions for unique institutional data, and select and integrate appropriate subject vocabularies into VIVO.

UF team members had national leadership roles from the project's earliest days. In the first year of the grant, the national implementation team was led by a UF librarian, who provided general implementation support, and a UF programmer, who provided national technical support. During the first year, the national implementation lead and technical implementation lead traveled to four of the collaborating institutions to assist with setup and implementation and held weekly phone meetings to answer questions and assist local implementations with roadblocks and issues. In the second year of the grant, as local implementations became increasingly self-sustaining, the national implementation lead shifted into a UF local implementation role. National implementation discussions continued on a weekly basis within a successful model of community-driven support.

At UF, as at each partner institution, there were local implementation and outreach teams. Local teams from each institution participated in weekly or bimonthly phone meetings on national implementation and outreach to discuss each institution's unique experience. These discussions were important for advancing the work of the national teams; the conversations identified shared data issues, an important topic when working toward a network of interlinked data. At UF, librarians served on a wide variety of teams, both national and local, and in many different roles. Those roles were primarily concentrated in implementation, ontology, and outreach and are covered below in detail.

Local Implementation Team

UF's local implementation team was responsible for setup and management of the VIVO system and ensuring researcher profiles were accurately populated. The composition of the teams varied greatly at each participating institution; at UF the implementation team was led out of the Marston Science Library and included one librarian serving as local implementation lead, the national implementation lead, and four grant-funded positions: one project assistant, one ontologist, and two programmers. Two Marston librarians also provided minimal implementation support. During the course of the project, implementation issues to discuss and address included the following:

- System administration, setup, backups, authentication, and firewalls;
- Scope of the local system (whether to include entire campus or segments of campus);
- Types of people to include (faculty, staff, students, volunteers, courtesy affiliates, alumni, etc.);
- Opt-in or opt-out requirements of the institution;
- Available local and external data;
- Depiction of organizational structure;
- Policy and governance;
- Stewardship of the data; and
- Testing of data pre- and postsystem upgrades.

As UF was a development site, our local implementation team was heavily involved in the national implementation effort. As a result the UF implementation team participated actively in testing application upgrades (identifying application and data-mapping issues) and provided feedback on usability and user-centered design. While each institution installed the same VIVO application, there were significant differences: in underlying software; in structure of available local data and subsequent mappings; and in the needs, policies, and expectations of the local community. These differences in implementation fed into overall application developments and improvements.

UF also had a data steward with the primary responsibility of mapping data to the local VIVO system. This position assisted in development of the national VIVO core ontology and was a member of the local implementation team with duties that included the following:

- Understanding each data source, including privacy issues;
- Verifying that data mappings were complete and accurate;
- Testing the source data against the requirements of VIVO; and
- Evaluating upgrades prior to implementation to verify data translation continued to be accurate.

Within the national community, the data steward identified issues within the VIVO core ontology and assisted in prioritizing the issues to be addressed in subsequent upgrades.

Local Outreach Team

Outreach to the University of Florida campus was spearheaded by liaison and subject specialist librarians, primarily at the Health Science Center Library and the Marston Science Library, with other main campus librarians joining in toward the end of the two-year grant period. Outreach activities were a logical place for librarian involvement given their expertise in instruction and the close professional relationships UF librarians are expected to develop and nurture with their clients. One UF librarian served as local outreach lead and was supported by a marketing coordinator (one grant-funded, full-time employee) and a team of approximately fifteen librarians.

Before the team could provide outreach to clients, including faculty and staff, they were provided with training on a number of fronts:

- How VIVO is different from other networking tools, with an emphasis on semantic technology and the ability to harvest information from authoritative sources;
- Benefits of VIVO use by faculty, which includes increasing research visibility, facilitating collaboration, and the potential for exporting data to curriculum vitae (CVs) or tenure and promotion packets;

- Benefits to the institution, including raising the visibility of the institution, using VIVO as a recruiting, grant-matchmaking, and reporting tool; and finally
- How to manually update records.

Outreach to clients generally took the form of presentations to various faculty groups. College-level faculty assemblies, departmental faculty meetings, and unit committee meetings (for example, a curriculum committee of a particular college or an executive committee for an institute or center) all became viable venues. The team worked from materials created by the marketing coordinator; these included short and long versions of a PowerPoint presentation, which could be adjusted for timing and content, as well as handouts. The marketing coordinator also designed materials that could be handed out to clients or posted throughout campus, including flyers, full-color posters, postcards, and table tents. A web-based evaluation/Q&A form was created so that librarians could record feedback from clients after each outreach session. The questions posed by clients helped the team hone their message and, in some cases, provided useful information to feed back to the development team. The VIVO website was updated to include FAQs based in part on the numerous questions the outreach team received during and after presentations.

Another vital activity performed by the outreach team was to help clients augment their VIVO profiles and troubleshoot any problems related to the profiles. Due to the fact that the VIVO harvester was a work in progress, and much of the information was being pulled from authoritative (but perhaps incomplete or incorrect sources), some clients had questions about missing or incorrect information appearing in their profiles. Examples included incorrect or missing publications, incomplete department or unit affiliation, or data that displayed incorrectly due to incorrect data mappings. Researchers tend to take such errors very seriously, and a deft hand was required to deal with clients. It was also important for the outreach team to have a thorough understanding of the harvesting process and schedule, as well as knowledge of who on the implementation team could help solve problems.

While harvesting existing information from authoritative data sources is a key feature of VIVO, some elements of the profile cannot be easily harvested from local or external sources. For this reason, the outreach team also solicited curriculum vitae from clients and manually entered some key elements to profiles, including educational background, previous positions, and research interests. Initially, only faculty from a select set of demonstration departments were asked for CVs, and librarians on the outreach team manually updated their profiles. Subsequently, asking for CVs became part of the general outreach message, and student workers on the project were available to perform the resulting data entry.

In addition to outreach to clients, the team also needed to provide outreach to the many librarians from throughout campus who were not initially part of the VIVO team. While VIVO outreach initially centered on getting buy-in from higher-level administrators and faculty in the health sciences and other sciences, toward the end of the project VIVO was rolled out to faculty across campus, including those from the arts, humanities, social sciences, education, and law. The subject specialist librarians who cover these units at UF had to undergo a similar training on using and updating VIVO, as well as the benefits of VIVO and how to publicize VIVO to their academic units.

Midway through the project period the outreach team led a town hall meeting to which all UF librarians and library staff were invited. The meeting introduced VIVO and featured testimonials from outreach team members who had worked closely with clients and also those who had presented on the project at the national level. These testimonials served to energize non–team members and helped them get a feel for the excitement and interest in VIVO both on and off campus. The outreach team displayed a number of posters on VIVO that had been presented at national conferences, described the training that would be made available to the librarians, and answered any questions that arose. Approximately seventy people attended, with representatives from most of the libraries on campus. This meeting laid the foundation for outreach throughout the entire Gainesville campus. Subsequently, outreach team members offered twelve training sessions, which were attended by approximately forty librarians from across the library system. A final support for campus librarians was the assignment of "VIVO partners." Each librarian had a designated VIVO partner who was their point of contact on the UF VIVO outreach team; VIVO partners answered follow-up questions on VIVO and were available to attend departmental meetings with other librarians. VIVO partners were rarely asked to visit departmental meetings, but the established support structure provided a mechanism for librarians to learn more about a new campus resource and feel more confident communicating its research value to the UF community.

CURRENT LIBRARY INVOLVEMENT

The library was integral to the development and implementation of VIVO, but after the grant-funding period ended, ongoing support was an appropriate fit with the CTSI's mission to foster collaboration. The UF libraries are periodically involved in areas of related support that have included the following:

- Identifying publications authored by all affiliated CTSI researchers for a given year;
- Performing literature searches to identify UF researchers who have published in areas of sex and gender differences or women's health and enhancing VIVO records to include subject-specific tags in these disciplines, publications, education, and more (in support of an NIH-funded outreach project);
- Examining VIVO publication data for the agricultural sciences as compared to the publication data collected within a unit-specific process;

- Working with VIVO representatives on the UF libraries data-management taskforce, with particular focus on the area of campus-wide ORCID implementation; and
- Discussing application of other areas of linked open data, such as BibFrame, and the possible overlap with VIVO.

CHALLENGES

Librarians working on VIVO encountered a number of challenges at all levels of the project. While specific challenges were dependent on both the team and the point in time of project development, generally speaking, challenges centered in two areas: skills and responsibilities, and dynamics and communication of teams. The challenges of the implementation and outreach teams have been discussed[5] but are included here as that relates to the library staff's grant effort.

Challenges related to skills and responsibilities were varied, but all library staff members were faced with learning curves. Members of all teams needed to be versed in the concepts and applications of the semantic web and linked open data. This knowledge was important when approaching local data providers and suggesting changes to VIVO data structure (implementation) and presenting at conferences (outreach). The implementation team members struggled with additional knowledge gaps, such as how to successfully approach local data providers for access to their institutional data, how to run SPARQL queries in order to extract or examine data, and how to continue to move forward within an environment of continuously changing expectation. Additionally, the implementation team was not affiliated with the CTSI and yet needed to understand the unique clinical and translational experience in order to implement a system that met their needs.

Challenges related to dynamics and communication of teams were due, in large part, to the diverse and geographically spread-out nature of the broader project team. Although there was a plethora of regular phone meetings and some in-person meetings across the national team, some librarians found it difficult to collaborate with people they did not know personally without the benefit of the nonverbal cues inherent with personal contact. The variety of communication channels available (phone calls, listservs, wikis, and other web-based project spaces) provided many opportunities for communication but were not always consistently used by team members. For librarians, interacting directly with developers was seen as a major benefit of the project. However, this involved overcoming some communication hurdles when librarians were unfamiliar with technical language and were unaccustomed to presenting on a project still in development. Communication and other challenges related to team dynamics improved throughout the course of the grant but were frustrating, particularly given that many members of the project team had never before been involved in this kind of cross-institutional collaboration.

OPPORTUNITIES

Although seven institutions took part in the VIVO project, this case study speaks to the individual and professional opportunities that were afforded the library faculty and staff involved in the project at the University of Florida. There were numerous opportunities for professional growth and development for all involved in the project. García-Milian and colleagues explored the VIVO experience through the context of the science of team science literature and enumerated a number of skills that were required for successful participation in the project, including strong communication and interpersonal skills, perseverance, ability to overcome obstacles, problem solving, agility, and leadership.[5] Many of these skills were gained over time through project work. While many of the outreach team members were experienced liaison librarians, a number of junior, nontenured faculty members were also part of the team. Through the VIVO project, these librarians gained extensive skills in marketing and publicity, developing and delivering effective presentations to varying levels of faculty/administration, project planning, and professional networking. Overall, even those librarians who were not part of the implementation team learned more about linked open data, the semantic web, and other technical applications. Because of the rapidly changing nature of the project and the need to work with a diverse, distributed group, it was important that the team be adaptable and comfortable with change—two attributes that the team became better at over time.

Aside from the incredible learning opportunity that VIVO presented to the faculty and staff who worked on the project, there were also numerous tangible benefits to team members. Most of the librarians in the Smathers Library system are tenured or on the tenure track, and as such, they are expected to perform research and produce scholarship through publications, presentations, grants, and other means. The VIVO project presented numerous venues for scholarly output. However, these opportunities were not limited to lines on a CV. The VIVO grant provided funding to attend scores of conferences, many of which were not on the UF librarians' typical conference circuit (for example, meetings of the west coast Medical Library Association chapter, the International Federation of Library Associations, the American Academy for the Advancement of Science, and the American Society for Human Genetics). Especially for the librarians who had not yet achieved tenure, being sent to conferences to present on VIVO allowed them to gain presentation experience, meet new colleagues, and extend their own professional networks.

On the UF campus, members of the outreach team benefited from enhanced professional relationships with their clients, as they presented at academic faculty departmental and college meetings. These presentations gave librarians the opportunity to discuss various library initiatives in addition to VIVO, such as open access, library workshops, and NIH public access policy compliance. For some academic units that had previously been reticent to have a librarian speak to their assembly, being part of an NIH grant seemed to provide more credence to the library, which facilitated its day-to-day work. Librarians also had numerous opportunities to present in university-wide research poster sessions, such as the annual Florida Genetics symposium hosted by the UF Genetics Institute, the Emerging Pathogens Institute Research Day, and the College of Medicine's Celebration of Research. Presenting the library's project next to those of academic faculty helped reinforce that library faculty are integrated into the university's research enterprise.

Finally, VIVO provides a number of institutional opportunities for UF and other participating institutions. VIVO exposes data to administrators, librarians, and funding agencies, assisting in the identification of campus support services, matching researchers with funding sources or collaborators, and connecting researchers with presentation and scholarship opportunities. As VIVO provides linked open data, which can be dynamically extracted and reused on websites and in multi-institutional searches, VIVO expands the institutional opportunities to build new and specialized networks. VIVO can also assist with institutional effort to disambiguate local researchers using ORCID identifiers.

At the national level, the CTSA consortium realized the value of research networking in general and VIVO in particular, as evidenced by their 2011 recommendation that "all CTSAs should encourage their institution(s) to implement research networking tool(s) institution-wide that utilize RDF triples and an ontology compatible with the VIVO ontology."[6] Pilot projects CTSAsearch[7] and Direct2Experts[8] make use of institutions' existing research networking tools (again, with an emphasis on semantic web technology and the VIVO ontology) to offer federated searching for people and expertise across the CTSA consortium. Just as CTS research relies on bridging disciplinary boundaries and working across the lines of college or department, it increasingly requires working on multi-institution projects with unique expertise represented at each institution. As such, the potential for federated searching of researchers' skills and knowledge across institutions provides opportunities for future collaboration, and VIVO has played a major role in encouraging interoperable infrastructure and vocabulary for research networking and discovery.

Beyond facilitating the discovery of individuals with certain expertise within the CTSA consortium, data from VIVO and other research networking systems can be used for more sophisticated network analysis. The VIVO platform itself includes built-in visualizations of each researcher's coauthor and coinvestigator networks, showing which individuals and groups a researcher works with most frequently. This type of network analysis has the potential to reveal broader patterns of collaboration in particular disciplines and changes in collaboration over time.[9] At UF's CTSI, network analysis has already been done (using VIVO data) to compare collaboration at the CTSI with other departments and institutes, identify individuals that serve as brokers across disciplines, see which resources are underutilized, and consider ways to change those networks that are not working optimally. Future social-network analysis work will focus on mapping knowledge networks, identifying characteristics of successful collaborators, and continuing to experiment with intervening in networks.

CONCLUSIONS

VIVO provided many excellent opportunities to UF librarians, and along the way there were many lessons learned.

- All people should have a clear understanding of the project and be encouraged to take ownership of their area of specialty, with the understanding that each individual serves the larger purpose.
- Communication between all parties must be set up as early and thoroughly as possible. This includes face-to-face meetings for local teams and online meetings for multi-institutional teams.
- Librarians' expertise and experience can contribute successfully to IT projects, particularly when knowledge of subject areas (such as CTS or agriculture) can help with translation between the field and the technology development. On the other side of that discussion, project managers should be knowledgeable of the skills and abilities of each team member to avoid misplaced duties and unnecessary frustration.
- Differences in team cultures can become roadblocks if not addressed through project management, communication, and responsibility discussions.
- Project management is not an inherent skill, and team members should be trained as early as possible. Project managers should develop clear lines of communication and a feasible plan. Always be cognizant of scope creep.
- Research networking and connecting potential collaborators is of interest across the country; librarians who get involved in research networking efforts can have a significant impact on their clinical and translational enterprise and broader institution.

NOTES

1. University of Florida Health Science Center. Health Science Center overview. 2015. https://ufhealth.org/health-science-center/overview. Accessed February 20, 2015.
2. University of Florida CTSI. About Clinical and Translational Science Institute at University of Florida. 2015. http://www.ctsi.ufl.edu/about/. Accessed February 20, 2015.
3. National Institutes of Health. Recovery Act 2009 Limited Competition: Enabling national networking of scientists and resource discovery (U24) 2009. http://grants.nih.gov/grants/guide/rfa-files/RFA-RR-09-009.html.
4. National Institutes of Health. Institutional Clinical and Translational Science Award (U54). 2007. http://grants.nih.gov/grants/guide/rfa-files/RFA-RM-08-002.html.
5. García-Milian R, Norton HF, Auten B, Davis VI, Holmes KL, Johnson M, Tennant MR. Librarians as part of cross-disciplinary, multi-institutional team projects: Experiences from the VIVO collaboration. *Sci Technol Libr.* 2013;32(2):160–75.

6. CTSA Consortium Executive and Steering Committee. Research networking recommendations. 2011. https://www.ctsacentral.org/best%20practices/research%20networking. Accessed February 20, 2015.

7. CTSA Consortium. CTSAsearch. http://research.icts.uiowa.edu/polyglot/ctsaSearch.jsp.

8. Weber GM, Barnett W, Conlon M, et al. Direct2Experts: A pilot national network to demonstrate interoperability among research-networking platforms. *J Am Med Inform Assoc.* 2011 Dec;18 Suppl 1:i157–60.

9. Newman MEJ. Coauthorship networks and patterns of scientific collaboration. *PNAS.* 2004 Apr;101 Suppl 1:5200–205.

10

Connecting Researchers

Designing a Networking App for Clinical Research Personnel

Christina N. Kalinger, Jean P. Shipman, and Roger A. Altizer Jr.

INSTITUTIONAL BACKGROUND

The University of Utah (UU) is located in Salt Lake City in the foothills of the beautiful Wasatch Mountains. It is Utah's only university with a health sciences academic center and is a Carnegie Mellon research extension, offering one hundred undergraduate and more than ninety graduate degrees to a student population of more than thirty-one thousand. UU has received more than $309 million in research and student aid funding from external sources and ranks fifteenth in the nation for faculty-awarded research.[1] It is also the home of biomedical informatics, with many long-standing data research databases, including the Utah Population Database (UPDB), Enterprise Data Warehouse, and a Utah all-payers insurance database. UU received Clinical and Translational Science Award (CTSA) funding in 2008; this funding was renewed 2013. The Eccles Health Sciences Library (EHSL) is home to the award's administrative center, the Center for Clinical and Translational Science (CCTS).

To further its goals to support and encourage clinical research, UU established a new department of population science in 2014 and, within it, a division of Health System Innovation and Research (HSIR). HSIR's mission is to promote the right care for every patient by enhancing the efficiency, value, and quality of care delivered by health-care systems and clinicians. To advance this goal, HSIR conducts outreach and provides support to many individuals across numerous disciplines and professions. Additionally, HSIR partners with the EHSL to identify the information needs of University of Utah researchers and to develop programs to meet those needs. EHSL's past efforts in outreach to the research community have been well documented and include the extensive review of the needs of UU researchers as part of its participation in the development of the My Research Assistant (MyRA) portal (see chapter 11). EHSL and HSIR have formed a mutually beneficial partnership and continue to reach out to researchers to identify remaining unmet needs.

PROJECT BACKGROUND

In its early months, HSIR hosted several informal sessions called "Breakfast, Lunch, and Dinner with HSIR." These sessions were intended to help the HSIR staff hear directly from UU researchers what specific tools or services could help them to be more effective in their research. One frequently expressed need was to break down departmental or disciplinary barriers and help researchers efficiently identify other researchers to facilitate connections and generate collaborations. This need is not unique to UU researchers; many universities have silos of expertise and experience challenges in communicating the breadth and depth of the research transpiring on their campus. While published research results often provide evidence of the knowledge being generated, this occurs only after the research has been completed to the point where it's ready for dissemination. Many researchers believe it would be highly beneficial to connect with others both inside their fields and in relevant or complementary disciplines prior to this point in the research life cycle.

This need has become even more apparent at UU with the Utah Science Technology and Research (USTAR) Initiative. USTAR is a program to encourage economic growth in Utah through funding research universities to support the creation of technology. The USTAR program was born from Utah's business community wishing to create a long-term investment in Utah's economic future. When the initiative passed the state legislature, millions of dollars were granted to the UU and other universities in Utah with the aim of funding research teams, building new research buildings, and recruiting faculty investigators. While this initiative provided a welcome influx of researchers and increase in research capability, the UU needed tools to help these researchers establish cross-departmental collaborations.

To attempt to solve this and other "connection" problems, the HSIR reached out to the Center for Medical Innovation (CMI). Founded in 2012, and housed on the garden level of EHSL, the CMI encourages innovation by serving as an information hub and connection point for the faculty, the staff, students, and the industry in the health sciences. It combines formal education programs, faculty and student project development, and support and facilitation of device development and commercialization. A new UU entity under the CMI is the Therapeutic Games and Apps Laboratory (The GApp Lab), which is also housed in the EHSL. The GApp Lab, established in January 2014, is comprised of graduate students in the Entertainment Arts and Engineering (EAE) program and partners with CMI and the EHSL to develop health-related games and apps. An innovation librarian and the director of

EHSL work closely with both the CMI and The GApp Lab to organize their outputs and intellectual processes and to support the innovation and educational programs.

HSIR contracted with The GApp Lab to develop a proof-of-concept tool to help connect researchers within and across disciplines based on areas of expertise and research interests. In conversations with HSIR personnel, the library director indicated that she had also seen a lot of demand for identifying research colleagues from other UU entities and shared some of the tools that exist commercially to assist with colleague connections and identifying expertise areas of authors. She encouraged HSIR and The GApp Lab to consider existing tools and UU faculty profile tools when designing the connection app.

PROJECT DESCRIPTION, PHASE ONE

A student team from the The GApp Lab was assembled like a collection of misfit Avengers. Our team included: (1) a producer who is in charge of keeping the vision of the project together and managing workloads, schedules, and anything that needs to be done; (2) an artist to create the art assets and oversee the visual design of the project; (3) an engineer who is the brain behind the code, ensuring that the developed features are both reasonable and functional; and (4) an additional producer who provides research assistance and examination of the academic and user theories behind the proposed solution to help inform the design. Our primary objective was to create a prototype of a research connection solution for HSIR using our collective game design skills, with the help of the EAE faculty and the EHSL.

After the design team was formed, our first step was to figure out exactly what we would be building to address the identified connection issue. To facilitate our brainstorming, we used a tool developed by our faculty advisor Roger Altizer called the Design Box. The Design Box is "a tool that encourages ideation and iterative pitching . . . [and] combines brainstorming/ideation, design, and pitching into a pedagogical tool that promotes team buy-in."[2] The Design Box is an easy-to-learn tool that identifies four aspects or walls a design must address: play/question/theory, audience, aesthetics, and technology. The play/question/theory wall highlights the specific mechanic, idea, or problem that the project must address. The audience wall identifies the intended user base or the project's target audience. The aesthetics wall covers the overall feeling for the project, highlighting the interactive content and the project's desired resulting user experience. The technology aspect forces one to ask which technology focuses of the system or tools will be applied to create the project. The team huddled for a session using Design Box to create the initial project pitch for HSIR; the rough Design Box is presented as figure 10.1.

We led off our initial design session by working on the play/question/theory wall. HSIR had expressed interest in a tool to help researchers connect, but we wanted to expand on this and address what we saw as a broader need—a clean, easy-to-use

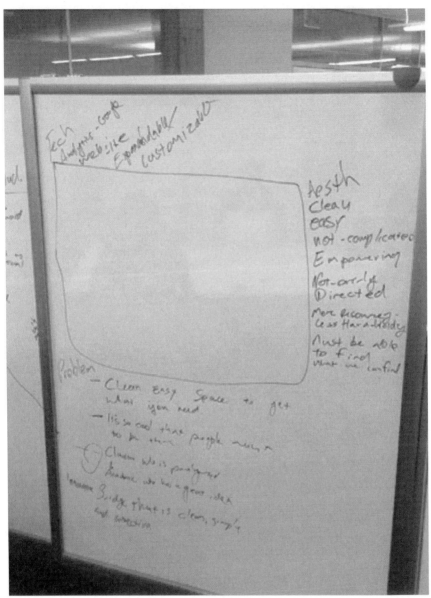

Figure 10.1.   The original Design Box for the project.

site a researcher can visit to identify and access not only collaborators but also all the resources needed during the research process. We determined that creation of this "one-stop connection shop" was truly the driving theory behind the project and would also address one of the needs identified during the MyRA project by the EHSL, as it functions to connect researchers early on in a project's life cycle. Our prototype would be a tool within a tool and would help researchers find both partners and other resources quickly and easily.

This concept also served to inform our aesthetic wall; we envisioned a look and feel that was simple yet empowering, enabling researchers to easily navigate the site and discover useful resources without a text-heavy interface cluttering the user experience. In terms of the audience, we identified two distinct groups: UU researchers and departments seeking collaborators within the institution and researchers who want to connect with individuals more suited to assist them in routine research operations. We also hoped the design would appeal to people external to UU who were looking for good examples of a sleek research navigation system.

When we came to the technology wall of our Design Box model, construction proved to be tricky. Were we developing for a mobile experience or something entirely different? While mobile technologies continue to gain a market share, we believe researchers still typically access research systems through the UU website on a personal computer or university-supplied workstation. Ultimately, we decided to craft a solution that utilized a website since we wanted to build a strong base for a tool that could be used to bring people or institutions together. But even with these parameters defined, where should we begin? The possibilities for a website-based tool are nearly endless.

Our breakthrough came when we began to consider existing models on the Internet where people connect with each other, spaces that are well known for their simple and easy-to-navigate user interfaces: dating websites and social media sites. The purpose of these sites is to connect potentially compatible strangers with similar interests—what better model for a researcher connection tool? While this gave us a good starting point, we didn't want to simply copy either dating sites or existing researcher tools when considering the user experience. This is where academic research came into play. We asked the innovation librarian which databases to use to find relevant peer-reviewed papers and studies on how adults use the Internet to network in order to help support our design decisions. For example, we researched current theories behind how social networking works with adults and learned that adult users may be less likely to use social media sites to make new connections.[3]

How this finding related to collaborations using technology, specifically communicating over the Internet, with medical professionals and researchers alike was unknown.[4] It told us something important about social media usage though: Adults rarely use their friends lists for professional networking on places such as Facebook. Most often, they'd use professional websites such as LinkedIn, but there is little room for research-oriented networking on these sites. It was often difficult to determine what field someone specialized in or if they'd been published, and if that information *was* available, it was often buried in favor of more common background information; for example, previous employers, institutions attended, and so forth. Given this limitation of typical professional networking sites, we determined that we needed a simplistic design to help researchers find relevant data to inspire collaborative relationships. The HSIR tool, we thought, should eliminate a lot of background information and focus on only the basics. Who are the researchers, what fields did they work in, what were their research interests, and where could you find their publications?

Once we had a basic design concept in place, we started thinking of other technologies we could use to make the connection process easier for users, helping them find resources as well as people. The topic of natural language processing (NLP) surfaced in the form of "chatbots," computer programs that are designed to simulate normal conversation among humans. Cleverbot[5] is one such program; it's one of the most long-lived chatbots and "learns" from all the input it is given to create increasingly realistic interactive experiences.

On the surface, this might not appear to have anything to do with a collaboration tool, but we had an idea. What if we used NLP, or a modified chatbot, to help direct researchers to key resources? Rather than requiring users to search a website to find research support resources, the chat program could potentially call on a keyword system to index various pages and function as an interactive search engine of sorts. That, combined with a minimal interface, could provide a straightforward experience for users of any skill level, no matter where they happened to be in their research process. We envisioned this use case: A user opens a browser and goes to a designated website. There, the user finds a few buttons highlighting major steps of a project life cycle (e.g., idea, design, implementation, evaluation, and dissemination), a link to HSIR, and a chat box with a prompt such as "How can I help?" The user types a question into the chat box, such as "How do I find funding?" The chatbot recognizes the keyword "funding" in its index and either asks a clarifying question or provides hyperlinks to locations on the website where the user could find relevant information.

After some good old-fashioned brainstorming and development of the general user story using Design Box, we concluded the design process with a simple market analysis: What current tools or programs exist, and how could we create something different that improved on them in some unique and important way? EHSL librarians were very helpful at this stage. Librarians met with our development team to walk us through existing licensed tools available to UU researchers, such as Unbound Medicine's Grapherence and a subset of Elsevier's SciVal Experts, and talked to us about the frequent requests for this type of resource by numerous individuals. In addition to learning about these tools, we created a document listing commercial or professionally related programs, no matter how little they seemed to have in common with the proposed design. For example, ResearchMatch is a system that matches researchers to study participants, with limited functionality and user base.[6] Then there's the ORCID system, an open-source tool that assigns a persistent ID number to researchers to help aggregate their publications and disambiguate their work from that of researchers with the same name.[7] We integrated relevant information into our plan, including the potential of integrating ORCID to populate researcher profiles, and presented our initial pitch to HSIR.

PROJECT DESCRIPTION, PHASE TWO

The design process in The GApp Lab is intentionally fluid and based on agile development, which allows for new research or information to influence final products in positive ways.

The benefits of our agile development philosophy became apparent when we presented our initial pitch to HSIR and received feedback that greatly impacted our original design. First, there was the difficulty of scoping the project and selecting a prototype design that worked for everyone. We had been excited at the prospect of using NLP to create an interactive system to link researchers with resources—human or otherwise—throughout the research life cycle, but HSIR requested that we limit the scope of this project specifically to the creation of a researcher networking tool. Additionally, we learned that there is an existing UU entity charged with website creation for the health sciences and that we did not have the proper authorizations to create a new website, which meant we had to drop that aspect of the project.

We also abandoned the idea of integrating ORCID profiles to populate the tool; while this initially seemed as if it might add value to our design, the project funders wanted a tool that could integrate with the existing UU Campus Information Services (CIS) system. CIS is a university-managed database of personal information linked to the unique ID number assigned to every UU employee, faculty member, and student, and HSIR wanted the team to use this, rather than ORCID, as a data source. Using UU IDs to link to CIS data would obviate the need for users to create a profile and manually enter personal data such as contact information. Using CIS would definitely involve a few extra steps in terms of data security but ultimately could serve to extend the tool to additional potential users, not only those at UU but also any other institution or group with a similar personnel database. As our primary goal was to deliver a tool that HSIR approved of and that could be used to achieving HSIR's goal of increased collaboration or connection, we had to incorporate this useful feedback into our design strategy. A prototype log-in screen using CIS credentials is presented in figure 10.2.

When we regrouped for another Design Box session, we reexamined every aspect of our model to figure out how to proceed. Our charge was now clear: HSIR expressed a desire specifically for a connection tool to help researchers identify potential collaborators in a more efficient and effective manner. Now that we knew the tool would focus only on connecting researchers based on topics of interest, we approached the rest of the project from a slightly different angle. We decided to retain the idea of basing our design on dating sites. We jokingly called the project "Tindr for researchers" or "Researchr" in order to remind ourselves that we had to

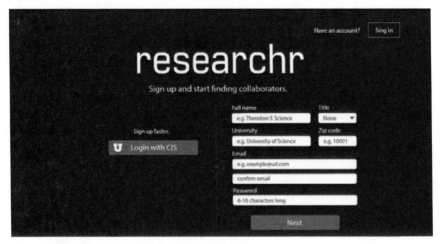

Figure 10.2.   Prototype log-in screen.

keep things simple. We kept the name "Researchr" throughout most of the project and named our final prototype "Colleague" once we had solidified most of the design and functionality.

Given our new, more tightly focused goal of creating a tool to match two compatible researchers together, we knew that representing shared topics of interest and fields of study of the researchers was essential. But how could we represent that in a sleek and uncluttered manner? It's not easy to take the words out of a design when there's a lot of information to parse. But our market analysis had provided numerous examples of websites where shared interests were buried in pages and pages of dense text, in effect requiring prospective partners to sort through resumes for potential collaborators. We knew we couldn't use NLP, because creation of the requisite tag and index system was too complex for the short amount of time allotted. During a meeting with the EHSL librarians about existing collaboration systems, the team programmer had an idea: Use word clouds. Data could easily be presented in word clouds, with the most common or most cited topics appearing in a larger font, making it simple to glance at a profile and quickly view the most important concepts in a given researcher's field of study. Figure 10.3 shows a mock-up of what this might have looked like from the design document, and figure 10.4 is the prototyped version.

This sounded like a great idea in theory, but it didn't work so well in practice. First, we discovered that the word-cloud solution created difficulties similar to those posed by NLP; it would be too time consuming to develop a tagging system or implement a plug-in that would be able to accurately identify research topics. Additionally, a word cloud can't precisely convey the experience or expertise at the level we required, and the generation of too many words created noise that undermined our desire to keep things clean and simple. To see the final design, refer to figure 10.5.

Ultimately, our research into dating applications strongly influenced our final design for Colleague. The bottom line was that it was essential to remove barriers for

Matching Page

Provide the researcher's name and university of residence.

Since it's not a dating thing there's no point in showing a picture, but we can use a word cloud of their research areas of interest to make it visually engaging while giving relevant study info.

If both researchers select yes for each other, the match will show up in their home pages.

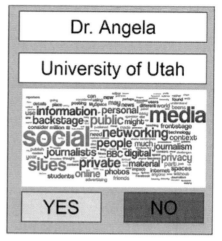

Figure 10.3. Word cloud mock-up in the design document.

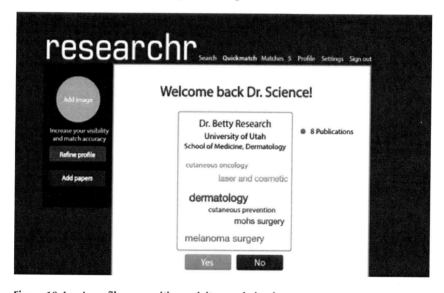

Figure 10.4. A profile page with specialty word cloud.

participation; in other words, we wanted to make it as easy as possible for researchers to navigate the tool and make effective use of Colleague. It had to be simple enough to integrate with an existing website (e.g., MyRA) but robust enough that it could stand on its own within existing HSIR web space. Additionally, when we designed this tool, we did not know where it would ultimately end up, since it was a prototype and a proof of concept.

Inspired by mobile dating apps, we settled on a fairly sparse user interface with only a few activities in order to minimize any distractions and avoid confusing the

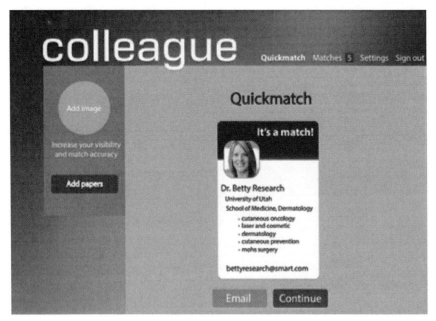

Figure 10.5.   Match screen presentation.

user. First, the user is invited to add professional publications to his or her profile in order for the system to index associated keywords or topics into a database. Once a researcher has created a profile, it's easy to access the match function, where he or she will see potential matches to other researchers, resulting from shared keywords or study types. The user can either confirm the match, at which point an e-mail form appears to facilitate contact, or reject the match, which results in another relevant researcher being presented. There is even a quick match option that automatically selects the closest match based on several topic commonalities.

Colleague also has a search function to help find matches based on specific subjects or narrow results. Once the user conducts a search, he or she is presented with a potential researcher match and that researcher's list of topics of expertise based on terms from the research profile. This data could, possibly in later editions of the tool, be added automatically once researchers link their publications to their profile or remain a manual addition—similar to what one would find when asked to list one's interests on a dating profile—and voilà, a simple tool that helps researchers quickly and easily find collaborators on a wide variety of topics. Figures 10.6 and 10.7 illustrate the final design concept.

LESSONS LEARNED

It's worth stating again that Colleague was designed and is presented here as a working prototype and not a finished product—it's meant to be both improved upon and

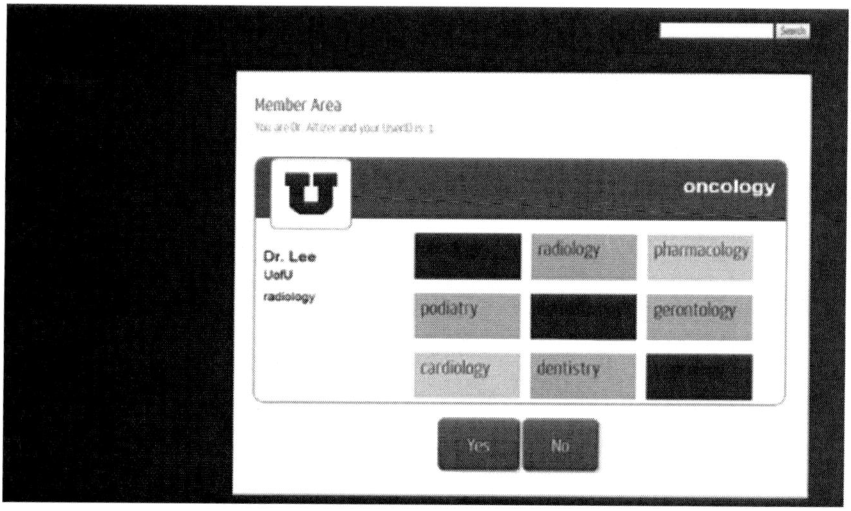

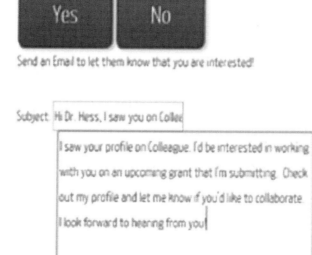

Figure 10.6. A grid of interests is presented with the match.

Send an Email to let them know that you are interested!

Subject: Hi Dr. Hess, I saw you on Colleague

I saw your profile on Colleague. I'd be interested in working with you on an upcoming grant that I'm submitting. Check out my profile and let me know if you'd like to collaborate. I look forward to hearing from you

Message

Send

Figure 10.7. Send an e-mail to initiate collaboration.

extensible. We had to accomplish a lot with limited resources and in a short time frame. We are a small group of students with limited experience in research and design, so there are bound to be overlooked preexisting systems or research that could have aided us immensely.

One of our biggest challenges is determining and demonstrating the potential impact of this tool. Web-traffic tracking and reports would only cover so much ground. How could we truly determine if Colleague could help researchers connect? The EHSL librarians would definitely have been useful in this regard given their role as a hub and connector for many different departments. They often know who is collaborating and where researchers' various interest areas may overlap as they work directly with a variety of researchers from all health sciences programs. They can expertly search the literature to identify what topics local researchers are publishing about and also use research networking tools or citation databases, such as SciVal and Scopus, to see clusters of related research publications. Another problem we face in the future of development is managing user expectations while encouraging use of our existing product. Not everyone wants or needs a simple tool such as this to find collaborators, but we want to encourage its use among all the populations we named as a potential audience or user base.

The pitfalls we encountered during this project were not unexpected or as numerous as they could have been, as our agile style permitted us to consider information from the EHSL librarians and feedback from HSIR and to adapt our design goals accordingly. We do recognize that additional resources would have enhanced our work. More time to complete a project is always desired; in this case, we were only funded for one semester to go from concept to working prototype, and we could have accomplished much more with a longer development cycle. For example, we could have improved existing features, including our keyword/tagging system and the visual design of the user interface. Additionally, if we'd had more programming power, perhaps we could have figured out a way to integrate UU IDs with the ORCID system to populate the research database with publications more efficiently.

Finally, improved communication with UU's public affairs and marketing unit and administration would have been beneficial, as we spent time planning a portion of the project that we had to abandon due to branding guidelines. Despite these challenges, we believe our prototype not only was successful but also shows potential for future growth or development. There are an endless number of systems this tool could be married to, including conference registration or abstract submission systems. For example, with slight modifications, Colleague could help conference attendees network before and after events or make it easier to locate contact information or presentation information postconference.

FUTURE

We began this project with the intent of building a prototype of an entire system to help researchers identify and use relevant resources in every step of the research life cycle. We adapted our goals and design based on research and input from HSIR (our funders), EHSL librarian collaborators, faculty mentors, and any other source of feedback we could get. Based on this feedback, we refined the design to the best of our ability and generated a proof-of-concept prototype.

Our funders from HSIR were pleased with the prototype that had been created, noting that it met the goals they had set for the project, and they decided to extend the project another semester. A new team of students from The GApp Lab will have a chance to take the tool from proof of concept to a stage where usability testing and iteration would be possible. Ultimately, that's the end result that every team hopes for—the ability to see their work continued to provide a foundation for a more solid experience. In this important regard, the HSIR tool was a success.

The partnership between The GApp Lab and the EHSL was also a success and was crucial to our project development. This collaboration provided us with access to professionals who were able to steer us in the right direction on more than one occasion and who were willing to lend their expertise to the design process throughout development.

We know that our partnership with the EHSL is one of the most important things that could have happened to us. Their assistance was evident in many forms, most notably the constant and incredibly useful information from the innovation librarian (IL). The IL regularly attended design meetings and recommended that we look into angles and research that we might have overlooked. If we had a question or needed information, she would get back to us quickly with all the sources we asked for. She also helped clarify the population we were developing for, ensuring that we understood the needs of our user base. Whatever we needed, whether it was answers or reassurance that we were moving in the right direction, the EHSL was there to support us. Good design is made even better when it's supported by extensive research, evidence, and theory, and we're happy that such a collaboration existed as part of our project.

From the EHSL viewpoint, being able to work so closely with The GApp Lab has enabled us to observe the intellectual processes employed to create therapeutic games and apps. We knew that we would be able to offer them assistance with their research to create the medical context of their products, but what we didn't realize was how much they would teach us about the need to capture the knowledge that was being generated and how the preservation of game parts or components is complex due to the number of different file formats involved. As a result, we have started capturing various game files each semester and have loaded them into e-channel (http://library. med.utah.edu/e-channel), a UU EHSL alternative publishing venue. We didn't realize the different areas of expertise needed to create an app, thus the interprofessional team of engineers, artists, producers, and research assistants. It has also been fun to share professional presentation and publishing opportunities and to discuss possibilities and venues with the students; this chapter illustrates one of the outputs of our joint efforts. The EHSL and The GApp Lab have mutually benefited from this close working partnership, and we have only just begun to explore the potential for future collaboration.

ACKNOWLEDGMENTS

We'd like to thank the following individuals for their valuable contributions to the Colleague Project: Kim Bowman, manager, HSIR; Tallie Casucci, innovation librarian, EHSL; Siddharth Gupta, engineer, The GApp Lab; Rachel Hess, director, HSIR; Katherine Marsh, artist, The GApp Lab; Travis Turner, producer, The GApp Lab; and Lauren Kirwan, administrative assistant, HSIR.

NOTES

1. University of Utah. Office of Budget and Institutional Analysis. http://www.obia.utah .edu/.

2. Altizer RA, Jr., Zagal JP. Designing inside the box or pitching practices in industry and education. Paper presented at Digital Games Research Association (DiGRA) conference; August 3–6, 2014; Snowbird, Utah. http://www.digra.org/wp-content/uploads/digital-library/digra2014_submission_134.pdf. Accessed December 5, 2014.

3. Subrahmanyam K, Reich SM, Warchter N, Espinoza G. Online and offline social networks: Use of social networking sites by emerging adults. *J Appl Dev Psychol.* 2008 Aug; 29(6):420–33, p. 426.

4. Kock N, Davidson R, Wazlawick R, Ocker R. E-collaboration: A look at past research and future challenges. *J Syst Inform Technol.* 2001 Jan;5(1):1–8.

5. Cleverbot. http://cleverbot.com/. Accessed December 5, 2014.

6. ResearchMatch. https://www.researchmatch.org/. Accessed December 5, 2014.

7. ORCID. ORCID: Connecting research and researchers. http://orcid.org/. Accessed December 5, 2014.

11

Librarians Partner with Translational Scientists

Life after My Research Assistant (MyRA)

Jean P. Shipman

INTRODUCTION

The University of Utah (UU) is nestled in the beautiful foothills of the Wasatch Mountains. It offers more than one hundred undergraduate programs and more than ninety graduate programs. It is the only health sciences academic center in the state of Utah with schools of medicine and dentistry and colleges of health, nursing, and pharmacy. The associated UU health-care system consists of four hospitals and ten community clinics. The UU was awarded a Clinical and Translational Science Award (CTSA) in 2008, which was reissued in 2013. This award is administered by the Utah Center for Clinical and Translational Science (CCTS). The CCTS consists of cores including biomedical informatics; clinical services; community outreach and collaboration; patient-centered outcomes research methods; recruitment, retention, and safety; research education, training, and career development; study design and biostatistics; and translational technologies and resources.

The administrative offices of the CCTS reside on the garden level of the Spencer S. Eccles Health Sciences Library (EHSL), the only health sciences academic library in the state of Utah. The EHSL is the MidContinental Regional Medical Library and the National Library of Medicine Training Center for the National Network of Libraries of Medicine. The EHSL is located in the center of the health sciences campus and is mainly a digital library of resources that houses an innovation center and fabrication laboratory, as well as the CCTS.

Due to the close proximity and the concurrent research support missions, the CCTS and the EHSL partnered to create My Research Assistant (MyRA) and fund a research concierge to support translational researchers.[1] MyRA is a portal containing information needed by new and experienced translational scientists at various stages of their research. It originated as a result of an extensive needs assessment that included conducting surveys, focus groups, and the deliberations of an appointed committee. MyRA included local and federal grant-related information as well as required sponsored program forms and processes. It was created via a partnership between the EHSL and the Department of Biomedical Informatics. This chapter reports on life after MyRA was released and how EHSL continues to meet the informational research needs of translational researchers and others at the UU.

MYRA'S IMPACT

The intent of this chapter is not to restate how MyRA was created[1] but rather to inform readers of the results of EHSL involvement in MyRA's formation, including discussion of the numerous partnerships and tools that have come about due to both MyRA and to the relationships we established during its creation. The key connector between the pre- and post-MyRA development days is that translational researchers still have a large number of information-related needs; many remain unaddressed even though they have been identified and documented. In reviewing the needs assessment document created through extensive interviews and surveys as part of MyRA's development,[2] it was apparent that many of the outlined needs remain unmet. Why? Because translational research is complex; there are many units on a health sciences academic campus that support translational research. It takes a lot of coordination of effort and time to develop tools and resources that meet various information needs. In order to tackle more of the needs we identified during MyRA's development, a research concierge was hired with combined funding from the CCTS and the EHSL. This individual was employed for one and a half years.

Research Concierge

One obvious need for all kinds of researchers is a place to go for answers to research-related questions, including how to obtain needed equipment, forms, and information on regulatory issues; where to publish research results for the most impact; what reporting requirements exist (what needs to be reported to whom and when, and what reports are due to which agencies, internally and externally, etc.); and how to effectively manage extramural funds and payrolls. Creating this one-stop shop that provides key guidance along the research life cycle was the primary goal behind MyRA. However, we quickly learned that researchers still want a personal contact to reach out to beyond any technological tools that are created—they still want to be able to talk to a person. Thus, a research concierge was hired that reported directly to the EHSL director and indirectly to the CCTS.

The idea emulates a hotel concierge: The research concierge could be asked questions that would either be answered immediately or triaged to the appropriate

UU unit or person. Over time and with experience, the research concierge would learn where expertise resides at the UU and could record this information so that others could consult a curated list of experts rather than having to rely on the concierge as an intermediary.

To fill the research concierge position (appendix 11.1), we hired a librarian with an interest in biomedical informatics and who was technologically savvy. He attended CCTS steering committee meetings along with the EHSL director and participated in CCTS administrative meetings. His web-development skills were quickly recognized, and he was asked to reinvent the CCTS website as a part of his responsibilities. He also led a lean training team that explored means for enabling translational researchers to easily request core resources and clinical trial support. He investigated different ideas for pulling together data from the various faculty profile systems offered by the UU. In addition, he explored the use of VIVO in order to link UU faculty with other researchers nationally. To address questions, an Ask MyRA e-mail chat feature was added to the CCTS website. Questions posed were analyzed in hopes of creating an FAQ document as well as a potential automated referral mechanism for themed questions.

The research concierge prepared monthly reports of his activities to share with the UU Office of the Vice President for Research and the EHSL director. These reports included statistics of the number of questions posed to the concierge as well as "Ask MyRA," a themed summation of the nature of the questions posed; the types of referrals made to others, including which units and individuals; and a dashboard reflecting trends over time. Also supplied were accomplishments achieved during each month and key meetings attended. Any additions made to the MyRA portal were recorded in these monthly reports, as were website-usage statistics and trends.

These reports documented the impact of the research concierge and provided indicators of additional services and resources desired by UU researchers. They also helped to illustrate the need for such items and helped to substantiate the existence of the MyRA research life-cycle one-stop-shop philosophy. Alas, the research concierge was so successful in this role that he was hired by one of the CTSA's partners to work in its research office.

Research Librarian

Discussions about whether or not to replace the research concierge position ensued. Due to the lack of funding, the CCTS decided it could no longer cofund the position. The EHSL then assessed its needs and pursued hiring a full-time, tenure-line research librarian rather than replacing the research concierge. The research librarian continues to support the CCTS but also assists with performing literature searches to meet the increasing demand and liaises with basic scientists, especially in genetics. A job description for this position is found in appendix 11.2.

The research librarian is active in instruction; classes "taught include "Publishing SMART," "Research Data-Management Sharing and Ownership," and "FURTHeR

Training" (a UU-developed search engine for anonymously identifying individuals for possible enrollment in clinical trials). The research librarian also offers one-on-one consultations—one key topic is assisting researchers with National Institutes of Health (NIH) public access policy compliance—and creates LibGuides on relevant topics such as research impact, information resources for researchers, protocols, NIH public access policy, and FURTHeR usage tips.

MYRA MOVES TO OFFICE OF SPONSORED PROGRAMS

As MyRA became better known and more widely used, questions were raised about its broader applicability and the value of hosting the site's content on a different platform for broader exposure. The UU Office of the Vice President for Research really liked the purpose and organizational structure and requested that MyRA be moved to a more UU-centric location in order to broaden its scope beyond CCTS personnel. As a result, MyRA became part of the Office of Sponsored Programs (OSP) website. The rationale was that many researchers need assistance throughout the research life cycle, not just those conducting translational science. Additionally, as many of MyRA's components originate within the OSP, hosting it on the OSP site would be a natural place for researchers to look for this information. This "rehoming" discussion took place simultaneously with the loss of CCTS funding for the research concierge.

In order to sustain MyRA's purpose and to enable it to have a broader scope, MyRA officially moved to the OSP website with a revised life-cycle look (figure 11.1). Some of the more clinical items were retained for a period of time on the CCTS website under a MyRA tab (this information has since been removed with a new CCTS website design). The history of MyRA was added to the new OSP website to reflect the growth of the concept over time.[3] Since the move, OSP has maintained and enhanced the life-cycle tool for more than three years.

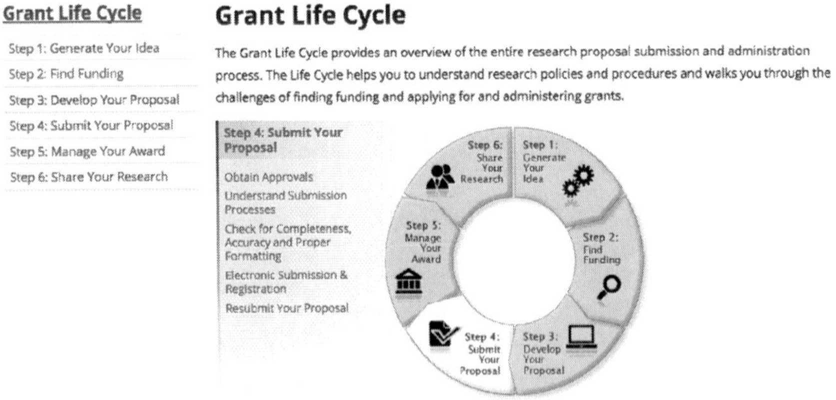
Grant Life Cycle
Step 1: Generate Your Idea
Step 2: Find Funding
Step 3: Develop Your Proposal
Step 4: Submit Your Proposal
Step 5: Manage Your Award
Step 6: Share Your Research
Grant Life Cycle
The Grant Life Cycle provides an overview of the entire research proposal submission and administration process. The Life Cycle helps you to understand research policies and procedures and walks you through the challenges of finding funding and applying for and administering grants.
Step 4: Submit Your Proposal
Obtain Approvals
Understand Submission Processes
Check for Completeness, Accuracy and Proper Formatting
Electronic Submission & Registration
Resubmit Your Proposal
Step 1: Generate Your Idea
Step 2: Find Funding
Step 3: Develop Your Proposal
Step 4: Submit Your Proposal
Step 5: Manage Your Award
Step 6: Share Your Research

Figure 11.1. OSP research life cycle.

The OSP research life cycle includes the same stepwise flow process we utilized on the original MyRA, including an overview of the grant life cycle, Generate Your Idea, Find Funding, Develop Your Proposal, Submit Your Proposal, Manage Your Award, and Share Your Research. Each individual step of the life cycle can be clicked to reveal additional resources, forms, tips, and techniques related to that particular part of the cycle.

The EHSL supplied much of the original life-cycle content, and both EHSL and UU's academic library, the J. Willard Marriott Library, are prominently featured in the last research life-cycle step, the Share Your Research section. Subsections, described below, deal with collecting and analyzing data, authoring and journal selection tips, publishing and peer review, archiving and preservation, and citation and metrics. This information continues to be updated by the two libraries in conjunction with the OSP.

Under Collecting and Analyzing Data, users can find information about how to gather data, including REDCap tutorials. The Clinical Services Center is also highlighted, as well as the Biomedical Informatics Core. Other CCTS cores are also emphasized, including the Study Design and Biostatistics Center, which provides biostatistician and epidemiologist expertise to many health sciences departments. Additionally, we provide links to statistical software licensed by the libraries, including SAS, SPSS, and Stata. Finally, a link to Databib gives users access to this registry of data repositories.

Featured in the Authoring and Journal Selection subsection is information about a UU writing center that assists with scientific writing, a technical writer directory, and training available related to publishing, including classes taught by the Research Administration Training Series (RATS) and by librarians. Two particular classes highlighted are "Publishing SMART: How to Make Your Article Visible" and "Getting Published: Responsible Authorship and Peer Review."

In the Publishing and Peer Review subsection, users learn how librarians can help them select journals in which to publish their research, as well as useful information about the publication peer-review process. Tips for how to alert the media about research results and subsequent publications are also provided. Authors are also encouraged to disseminate their research results via scholarly websites; techniques for doing so are shared in this subsection.

The Archiving and Preservation section provides information about open science and public policy related to research publications, such as NIH and National Science Foundation (NSF) public access policies. Links to many scholarly communication websites and useful tools such as SHERPA/RoMEO, JULIET, local and national databanks, and full-text article repositories are provided in this section.

Under Citation and Metrics, one can find details about citing requirements for major funding sources, as well as a LibGuide about the various bibliometric tools available to measure and quantify the impact of research. Here one can learn the difference between the Eigenfactor and the h-index, as well as understand how to collect citation counts for published journal articles.

Ask MyRA Question Summary

The Ask MyRA question feature is still monitored by EHSL librarians who answer incoming questions or triage them to content experts as appropriate. This feature has been revised to include a drop-down menu of choices that attempt to categorize the question being posed. The choices roughly match the life-cycle steps but are more specific and include Generating Ideas, Designing a Study, Finding Funding, Finding Equipment and Facilities, Finding Expertise, Writing Grants, Obtaining Study Approval from the Institutional Review Board (IRB) or OSP, Performing the Study, Analyzing Data, Reporting and Publishing, and Other. Links to this service appear on the CCTS and the Office of the Vice President for Research websites, as well as on various pages on the OSP website.

We receive around sixty questions per year requiring about twenty-eight manpower hours, or roughly half an hour per question. This reflects both the time to answer the question or interact directly with the patron and the time needed to do the requisite research. Most questions we receive center on the availability and location of needed resources such as equipment, statistician assistance, desired templates (e.g., grant writing, consultant, and data management), data-storage repositories, and software (e.g., REDCap and Qualtrics). Many questions also deal with IRB approval issues and NIH public access policy compliance. Other requests include the amount of UU extramural funding received per fiscal year, recommendations for needed collaborators and partners, and troubleshooting grant application glitches. Finally, we receive requests for help with literature searching for grant submissions.

BIRTH OF RISE: RESEARCH INFORMATION SERVICES

As we started working more with the CCTS cores, we quickly realized that our information services targeted for researchers could be considered a core, even though, unlike other cores, our family of services is free and not cost recovered. We contacted the then director of health sciences research and discussed the possibility with him. He quickly approved our inclusion as a core but recommended that we clearly present any available services in a manner meaningful to researchers—in short, drop the library jargon that often creeps into our service descriptions.

A blanket term for referring to the library core was needed and thus we birthed RISe—an acronym for the EHSL's Research Information Services. We added RISe to the EHSL website, as well as to the health sciences cores site (which was later moved to the university cores site).[4] The process of creating our cores page cemented our realization that we do offer a lot to researchers and our services are essential to their ability to complete their research, especially to disseminate their results. Figure 11.2 shows our entry on the cores page.

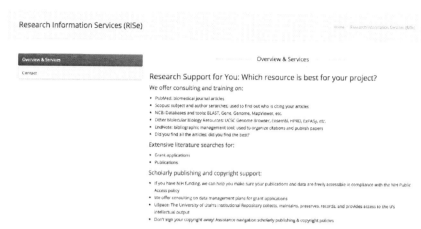

Figure 11.2. RISe entry on cores site.

CROSS-UNIVERSITY RESEARCH ASSISTANCE

Data-Management Plan Toolkit

With the advent of data-management plan requirements for federal grant recipients, which would particularly affect UU researchers receiving NIH and NSF funding, the Marriott Library and the EHSL partnered to determine how the UU libraries could best support researchers in writing their plans. A data-management task force was formed with members from both libraries, as well as information technology staff. We conducted a review of what other institutions were doing to support researchers in writing and did an environmental scan of electronic laboratory notebook software. A pilot project with a willing faculty member helped us identify questions that might arise and determine what kind of information was needed to formulate a data plan. These activities resulted in a white paper for internal use in which we recommended creation of a toolkit including templates for researchers to use to fulfill the data plan requirement depending upon their funding source. The toolkit is currently in use and continues to be updated and refined. Additionally, a campus data-management group was formed in 2014 to reassess and address the needs of researchers for data-management support.

Grant Writing and Research Support

In 2014, the UU Office of the Vice President for Research asked the Marriott Library to house grant-writing personnel. The library agreed and, from a desire to do more than just provide space to grant writers, formed a joint committee to provide additional support to faculty researchers. Cochaired by librarians from the Marriott Library and from EHSL, the committee is comprised of librarians from all three UU libraries. Their overarching goal was to increase the number of grants written by UU faculty. The charge to this joint committee included the following elements:

- Develop and maintain an online guide that contains information for finding grants in all subject areas, with easy access to NIH and NSF webinars and training materials.
- Create a website with links to descriptions of successful grants.
- Work closely with Technology and Venture Commercialization (TVC) and OSP to further develop a robust and sustainable patent searching program.
- Increase capacity for statistics support for central campus.
- Build an existing literature search service to increase capacity for all disciplines.
- Provide assistance with writing data-management plans.
- Work with the vice president for research and OSP to complement the training and workshops they offer to assist faculty applying for grants.
- Develop an on-demand, comprehensive literature search service for the Marriott Library.

The joint committee completed its work in late 2014, accomplishing most of its charge and, in the future, will be assessing how much use the new services and tools receive.

Library Involvement with University-Wide Research Committees

As with any large university, many committees and groups exist to help further research at the institution. It has taken several years to learn about the different groups and, more importantly, to earn a seat at their tables. The following is a list of committees on which EHSL librarians either are currently serving or have participated in the past. We recommend that librarians investigate which university committees might be receptive to having a librarian join their work and volunteer to serve. We found that it was not difficult to get added once we requested a seat at the table; often it was just an oversight about including a librarian. Our contributions have been well received, and our presence adds value to these committees: Our skills in quickly being able to identify and organize past evidence to contribute to future research is appreciated, as are our abilities to organize both content and people.

Research Advisory Council (RAC)

This group of health-sciences campus research administrators and researchers meets monthly to discuss research priorities in the health sciences.

CCTS Steering Committee

This committee meets every other month and is comprised of the CCTS codirectors, the heads of the eight cores, and UU health sciences leaders. The director of the EHSL also is a representative. The committee discusses approaches to addressing CTSA requirements, developing proposals, providing directions for the CCTS, and discussing means of integrating the CTSA partners.

University Research Portfolio

This group of individuals is responsible for setting priorities and initiatives and for allocating funding to improve technology, especially innovative technology, at the UU to address the advanced needs of researchers. There are representatives from various colleges and schools as well as the university information technology unit and the UU Office of the Vice President for Research, as well as members from both the EHSL and Marriott Library.

Research Deans Meeting

Under the direction of the UU Office of the Vice President for Research, deans, associate deans, and assistant deans overseeing research in their schools and colleges across campus meet monthly to discuss issues related to conducting research at the UU.

Campus Data Management

This is a committee composed of representatives from the EHSL, the Marriott Library, the Quinney Law Library, information technology, the Center for High Performance Computing, the Office of Sponsored Programs, and the UU Office of the Vice President for Research. Its charge is to development mechanisms to help faculty members manage their data to meet NIH, NSF, and other funding agency requirements. The ultimate goal is to inform the faculty of the UU's stand on data management and its guidance not only to meet funding requirements but also to enable faculty to be recognized for their research contributions, as well as get credit for promotion and tenure purposes. The group would like to assign criteria to state what and how data will be curated and prioritized for preserving over time. The group also educates the faculty about available data repositories both locally and nationally and how to effectively cite stored data to add to faculty recognition, and thus impact. Identifying permanent funding sources for data storage is another key goal of this group.

CHALLENGES FACED

Not surprisingly, we faced many challenges both in the implementation of MyRA and in our life beyond it. These challenges center on financial support, ownership, clarity of roles and responsibilities, and sustainability. As mentioned earlier, research within a university is a large enterprise with many people involved. Communications can also be challenging—we frequently encounter researchers working in information silos who are often unaware of the resources, services, colleagues, and facilities that are available to them.

While everyone agreed that something such as MyRA was needed, where it should reside was ultimately brought into question. Understandably, the UU Office of the Vice President for Research wanted to avoid duplicate effort in creating this or similar resources and wanted to ensure that correct information was being released about grant administration and regulatory compliance issues. They wanted this information to be both accurate and timely. The EHSL was not interested in duplicating work either and had intended to link to already-existing materials available from the UU Office of the Vice President for Research and OSP. Transferring the MyRA life-cycle concept to the OSP seemed a reasonable thing to do; in retrospect, we should have considered a partnership with these two offices when MyRA was created. The development of MyRA through the CCTS resulted from its inclusion in the CTSA proposal as a deliverable, but it was not funded when the CTSA was ultimately awarded. Thus, its initial focus was for translational research and not all researchers. We recommend that those starting out on a MyRA-like project consider all potential parties at the beginning and solicit their input and assistance. A more robust tool is definitely more advantageous to a university that must address all kinds of researcher needs.

Funding is another challenge that we faced. As stated above, there was no funding set aside in the final CTSA for the MyRA deliverable, yet everyone wanted it to be developed and had high hopes for its potential. While ideas were numerous and MyRA was often reported to be better than sliced bread, without appropriate funding, its development was cobbled together through the efforts of many individuals that served on a development committee. We received initial funding from the MidContinental Region, National Network of Libraries of Medicine; this helped to support the core technological infrastructure for MyRA. This funding supported development of a plain-vanilla HTML version that we could share with others desiring a similar tool, as well as a more robust version 2.0 MyRA framework that used Drupal and Alfresco. More funding would have enabled the entire vision for MyRA to have been created, including various researchers' personas that would push needed information at the right time to researchers based on the appropriate level of experience. Again, similar to MyRA, everyone loved the idea of a research concierge, but limited CCTS funding required the CCTS to discontinue its support of the position. Additional funding would have secured the position of the research concierge beyond the time it was supported.

Finally, sustainability is another challenge. Once we'd created the first several versions of MyRA, there was not a long-term plan for how to sustain further development and migrate to the new systems that inevitably appear over time. By transferring maintenance of the site to the OSP, there was some guarantee that MyRA would live on in some manner and that it would be updated through that office's staff.

Indirect research costs could help to sustain future site development and provide the needed personnel support. Just like grants, tools that support grant writers, administrators, and researchers need to have a sustainability plan established at the beginning to ensure that development efforts are not short term or in vain.

FUTURE

OSP Grant Life-Cycle Updates

Due to the changing nature of research and associated regulations and protocols, the OSP grant life-cycle tool will need to be continually updated. We work with the OSP, the UU Office of the Vice President for Research, and the Marriott Library to continue to refine and update the grant life cycle with relevant tools, forms, documents, and news. We also plan to pursue grant funding to implement many of the originally desired features of MyRA as envisioned in the MyRA white paper.[3]

Systematic Reviews Librarian

The EHSL receives an increasing number of requests to assist with systematic reviews. To meet this growing demand, we hope to fund a position for a systematic reviews librarian in the near future. This librarian will assist teams with discovering, reviewing, and analyzing the literature for evidence in support of establishing treatment consensus, a variety of types of interventions, and research protocols, and to aid cost-effectiveness and outcomes research. We envision this librarian will work closely with our CCTS, including teaching in the master of science in clinical investigation core courses and our Pharmacotherapy Outcomes Research Center (PORC). Some services of such an individual could even become a rechargeable core: Being able to charge for expert librarian services would help to build a financially sustainable model for a research librarian position.

E-channel

The EHSL has developed a new platform for disseminating the results of innovative research called e-channel (http://library.med.utah.edu/e-channel). It was released in March 2015, and content is being added frequently. E-channel is an interactive platform designed to capture and disseminate the creative output of innovators in all disciplines but particularly the health sciences. E-channel provides a forum for sharing process improvements, new technologies, brainstormed ideas, digital therapeutics (health applications and games), videos, and many other innovations. This multimedia portal enables the transfer of innovative ideas regardless of format and at various stages of creation and implementation. A unique feature of this platform is that it provides a venue for researchers to share their failures. Failures are important in innovation as others can learn from them and not replicate similar mistakes. However, to date, there has not been an outlet for disseminating information about failures. E-channel provides such an outlet: "This eclectic hub offers a venue for innovators and researchers to share their results, receive recognition, and contribute to their scholarly disciplines, while also ensuring that others can build on the work reflected."[5]

Researchers seeking a quick and convenient platform from which to disseminate their results or who wish to use a nontraditional, multimedia means to share their research may opt to use e-channel as an alternative distribution venue. We encourage others from outside the UU to contribute to e-channel by contacting us or completing forms provided on the platform in order to provide a rich forum of content that showcases innovative research. As e-channel becomes more globally recognized and used, we will be monitoring different metrics, such as hit rates, citation inclusion, and qualitative comments received to determine its success.

CONCLUSION

While this chapter has expressed the many ways the EHSL has worked to help researchers be successful, it is clear that our work will never be done; research is evolving and new needs are constantly surfacing. With the rapid pace of research translation, and as financial support for research has diminished in the last decade, we anticipate increased needs for information to be available at researcher's fingertips and in a manner that can be easily synthesized and digested. As more regulatory and administrative requirements are placed on researchers, they have less time to scan the literature or to share their results. There is a need for e-tools to be generated that can reduce administrative burden or streamline aspects of the research life cycle to save researchers' time and energy for their research. This continual demand for increasingly precise information at the point of need, in the format required, and in a timely manner will challenge information professionals in the future.

As research transpires across disciplines, there will need to be effective means of identifying research partners and collaborations, not only locally but also globally. Networking and expertise identification tools are just one example; please refer to chapter 10 in this book for a description of a prototype tool created at the UU to address this connection need.

Finally, librarians can increase the research standings of their institutions by becoming embedded partners with all kinds of researchers. Librarians should investigate ways to use their talents, expertise, and organizational skills to assist research teams in being more efficient and productive. The challenge to manage information that arises in research and help in translating it to the patient's bedside can be ours if we rise to the occasion and encourage others to see that we can add significant value to research teams.

APPENDIX 1:
RESEARCH CONCIERGE POSITION DESCRIPTION

Research Concierge
Position Description
March 20, 2012
Position Overview: A twelve-month, non-tenure-track research associate position that primarily collaborates and lends support to researchers, especially those affiliated with the CCTS and/or those doing clinical research.

Reports to: Spencer S. Eccles Health Sciences Library director and CCTS administration.

Specific Duties

- Schedule and track researcher consultations with CCTS cores and specialists.
- Monitor outcomes of consultations (e.g., number of grants received, funding received, and qualitative differences consulting made).
- Provide linkages between experts, mentors, and collaborators and researchers.
- Inform researchers of clinical trial information, registries, and regulations; maintain an inventory of CCTS-related clinical trials.
- Track CTSA partnerships with community organizations and players.
- Provide orientations for new faculty and researchers.
- Offer trainings on using collaborative work spaces, FURTHeR, and other relevant research databases; schedule trainings with special trainers as needed.
- Maintain calendar regarding training opportunities for researchers for all CTSA partners.
- Educate researchers about NIH, NSF, and other funding and local (institutional repository) compliance requirements, especially regarding publications and data.
- Maintain MyRA portal: collect and update its content and add new features.
- Monitor developments in social media, and apply relevant technologies to virtual collaborative CTSA spaces.
- Create and manage promotional materials about MyRA services and content.
- Collect evaluative feedback information for continuous improvement.
- Collaborate with other CTSA awardees to share knowledge, create tools, and develop partnerships; evaluate new tools.
- Maintain knowledge of CTSA trends and initiatives; build bridges with other CTSA institutions.
- Participate in CTSA regional and national consortia, and provide information and training support when possible.
- Serve on CCTS and CTSA and other university committees as appointed.

- Disseminate results of efforts through professional channels, including presentations and publications; be active in related professional organizations.
- Apply for and administer received extramural funding.

Required Qualifications

- Demonstrated knowledge of research process and funders
- Excellent interpersonal and communication skills
- Graduate degree in relevant discipline; for example, information science, basic sciences, clinical sciences, and so forth
- Evidence of excellent organization and problem-solving skills
- Demonstrated knowledge of Drupal and Alfresco software

Preferred Qualifications

- Evidence of extramural funding support
- Knowledge of evidence-based health sciences practices and resources
- Evidence of instructional course design and delivery experience
- Demonstrated familiarity with social media and its application to research
- Evidence of collaborative partnership and support experience
- Knowledge of array of research dissemination venues

APPENDIX 2:
RESEARCH LIBRARIAN POSITION DESCRIPTION

The faculty and staff of the Spencer S. Eccles Health Sciences Library at the University of Utah invite applications for a research librarian. The research librarian reports directly to the associate director for education and research and is responsible for supporting clinical and bench science biomedical researchers through reference, literature searching, outreach, and education. Primary domains for the research librarian's outreach and education are biomedical scholarly communication, grant cycles and compliance responsibilities, data-management planning, and research impact measurement. Depending on the qualifications and interest of the successful candidate, the research librarian may be embedded within the health sciences campus. Candidates with bench research experience and outgoing personalities are particularly sought. Other duties may be assigned. This position is a full-time, tenure-track faculty position. All librarians are expected to contribute to the profession through service, scholarship, outreach, and mentoring.

The mission of the Spencer S. Eccles Health Sciences Library is to advance and transform education, research, and health care through dynamic technologies, evidence application, and collaborative partnerships. The library contributes to the success of health professionals, students, researchers, and the community. The library is recognized locally and nationally as a leader of intellectual exploration and as a catalyst for innovative discovery. The University of Utah Health Sciences Center is known for cutting-edge research, particularly in genetics and biomedical informatics, and its Center for Clinical and Translational Science was refunded by the NIH in 2013. Health services research, personalized health care, population health, and innovation are new key research areas.

The Spencer S. Eccles Health Sciences Library (http://library.med.utah.edu) serves University of Utah Health Care, the Intermountain West's only academic health sciences center, including the schools of medicine and dentistry and the colleges of nursing, pharmacy, and health as well as the university hospitals and clinics. The library also serves as headquarters for the National Network of Libraries of Medicine, MidContinental Region, and the National Library of Medicine Training Center. It is a member of the Utah Academic Library Consortium, the Medical Library Association, the Association of Academic Health Sciences Libraries, and the Association of Research Libraries.

Required Qualifications

- Graduate degree from an ALA-accredited library school or other relevant accredited graduate degree
- Flexibility and adaptability for work in a fast-paced, changing environment
- Excellent interpersonal and communication skills
- Ability to work as a team member and independently
- Commitment to diversity in the workplace and community
- Willingness to seek membership in the Academy of Health Information Professionals (AHIP)

Preferred Qualifications

- Bachelor's or advanced degree in basic sciences or health-related field
- Bench science, pharmacy, or clinical research experience
- Previous professional work experience within health-sciences libraries
- Experience with evidence-based information retrieval and in-depth literature searching
- Knowledge of biomedical information resources, data management, and traditional and alternative research impact measurement tools
- Experience providing instruction in an academic setting
- Awareness of scholarly communication issues within the health sciences
- Demonstrated organizational and problem-solving skills
- Familiarity with emerging and established technologies, including mobile devices
- Sense of humor and outgoing personality

NOTES

1. Reich M, Shipman JP, Narus SP, et al. Assessing clinical researchers' information needs to create responsive portals and tools: My Research Assistant (MyRA) at the University of Utah—A case study. *J Med Libr Assoc*. 2013;101(1):4–11. doi:10.3163/1536-5050.101.1.002.

2. MyRA needs assessment report. University of Utah Office of Sponsored Programs. http://osp.utah.edu/about/myra.php. Updated December 29, 2014. Accessed January 19, 2015.

3. MyRA white paper. University of Utah Office of Sponsored Programs. http://osp.utah.edu/about/myra.php. Updated December 29, 2014. Accessed January 19, 2015.

4. University of Utah. HSC cores research facility. 2013. http://www.cores.utah.edu/?page_id=3703. Accessed January 19, 2015.

5. E-channel. University of Utah Spencer S. Eccles Health Sciences Library. http://library.med.utah.edu/echannel. Updated January 14, 2015. Accessed January 19, 2015.

12

The Role of the Library in Public Access Policy Compliance

Emily S. Mazure and Patricia L. Thibodeau

INTRODUCTION TO DUKE MEDICINE
AND THE RESEARCH ENVIRONMENT

Duke University in Durham, North Carolina, has a robust research enterprise. It ranked as the seventh-largest research university in 2012 with $1.01 billion in research expenditures[1] and has been consistently in the top ten since 2007, receiving more than $371 million from the National Institutes of Health (NIH) in 2014 (twelfth in terms of all NIH funding mechanisms).[2] The medical center (academic and research) has almost ten thousand full-time employees.[3] In 2013, there were more than four thousand active studies in the clinical research units, with 30 percent funded by the federal government, 30 percent by industry, and the rest through nonprofit foundations and internal funding.[4] In 2014 the *U.S. News & World Report* ranked Duke among the top ten medical schools, and five specialty-education programs ranked among the top ten.[5]

Duke University received one of the first Clinical and Translational Science Awards (CTSA) in October 2006, followed by a renewal in 2013. Duke Medicine is the administrative home to the CTSA. It consists of the Duke University Health System (including three hospitals), the School of Medicine (clinical and basic sciences), and the School of Nursing, all part of the research enterprise. There are 1,899 faculty members in the clinical program, 208 in the basic sciences, and 89 in the School of Nursing. Duke Medicine houses twenty-one basic science and clinical departments along with numerous centers and institutes. Like many other institutions, Duke used CTSA funds to support and further research programs by centralizing expertise in biostatistics and regulatory affairs, accelerating the pace of laboratory-based research into early-phase clinical trials, offering tools for managing and sharing data, and training researchers in translational medicine.

Duke Medicine established the Duke Translational Medicine Institute (DTMI) to house CTSA grant activities. This also brought together various research groups and service units on the medical campus such as the Duke Clinical Research Institute and a thirty-bed research service. DTMI was charged with ensuring that the infrastructure, resources, and training were in place to facilitate translating ideas into innovations and ultimately into improved health. DTMI established new tools and services and provided funding for specific projects. In addition to enhancing extant activities and funding new projects, DTMI garnered funding through other federal agencies and private sources to further expand Duke's research activities.

As part of the DTMI focus on infrastructure, the Duke Office of Clinical Research (DOCR) was created to provide more central oversight, expertise, training, and data management for the clinical research community and to reduce costs by sharing centrally managed expertise.[4] After a few iterations, clinical research was structured around clinical research units (CRUs) that provide oversight for any clinical research where Duke is the investigative site. The seventeen CRUs are organized around clinical service areas (such as children's and heart) as well as established research centers.[5] Each CRU has a director and managers for research practices and financial practices. This structure addresses funder requirements, federal regulations, and compliance issues as well as the actual conduct of the research.

The Medical Center Library and Archives serves all of Duke Medicine, from the research enterprise to educational programs and clinical care. Faculty members play multiple roles and are often researchers as well as clinicians and educators. While faculty members often turn to the library in these latter roles, the library was interested in strengthening its support of the research enterprise from clinical to basic sciences. When the first CTSA funds was awarded, the library director joined the bioinformatics planning team, but the team's focus on specific research tools and services did not translate to a role within the larger, complex award environment. In the meantime, librarians reached out to research units trying to support data needs, referred people to the newly coordinated research activities and tools, and continued to seek out opportunities to engage. One of the most successful opportunities to become involved in the research enterprise came about due to the implementation and enforcement of the NIH public access policy.

THE NIH PUBLIC ACCESS POLICY

In 2015, the NIH had an annual budget of $30.3 billion for medical research; more than 80 percent of this was distributed among more than three hundred thousand researchers.[6] Results of the research that is completed using this funding is eventually reported in peer-reviewed articles and published in scientific journals. Most of these journals require paid subscriptions to access their content; consequently, people without subscriptions, including NIH personnel and other scientists, might not have access to the products of federal funding. In 2005, NIH began to develop a policy to address this issue. The initial public access policy[7] had three aims:

1. *Archive.* A central collection of NIH-funded research publications preserves vital published research findings for years to come.
2. *Advance.* The archive is an information resource for scientists to research publications and for NIH to better manage its entire research investment.
3. *Access.* The archive makes available to the public research publications resulting from NIH-funded research.

In the course of developing the final version of the policy, NIH sought input from stakeholders, including the general public. In addition to advancing scientific discovery, the two most common reasons given for support of the policy were the potential benefits to patients and families and the right of American taxpayers to publications resulting from NIH funding.[7] In the notice of final policy, the policy's aims were broadened and included making "the publications of NIH-funded research more accessible to and searchable for the public, health-care providers, educators, and scientists."[8]

The final NIH public access policy requires all peer-reviewed articles, accepted for publication on or after April 7, 2008, that arose directly from NIH funding, to be made publicly available via PubMed Central (PMC) within twelve months of publication. Principal investigators (PIs) and authors need to take several steps to ensure compliance:

• They need to track which of their peer-reviewed articles are NIH funded and provide notice to the publisher at the time of submission of the funding of the requirement to submit to PMC.
• If their paper will not be published in a PMC journal (a journal that makes its contents available in PMC), the PI/authors need to ensure the final, peer-reviewed manuscript of their article is deposited to PMC. Sometimes the journal/publisher will submit this manuscript to the NIH Manuscript Submission System (NIHMS) or directly into PMC, but often the authors/PIs will need to submit it themselves.
• Any articles submitted to NIHMS will require two approvals, which the designated author will need to be aware of and respond to before the article will be compliant.
• Finally, PIs are responsible for ensuring all peer-reviewed research articles resulting from their grants are compliant with the public access policy.

When NIH first released the public access policy in 2005, submission to PMC was not mandatory; rather, investigators were "requested to submit an electronic version of the author's final manuscript upon acceptance for publication."[8] Neither publishers nor authors were prepared to comply, and submission rates reflected this. From

May 2005 to 2007, only 19 percent of the articles subject to the policy were submitted to PubMed Central. Of those, the majority (12 percent) were final published articles deposited by publishers, and another 7 percent were manuscripts submitted by authors or journals on behalf of authors.[7] Clearly, only a small proportion of the articles that fell under the policy were actually added to PMC by authors/investigators. Additionally, many submitted articles never cleared the various quality-assurance stages required before final deposit in PMC. Many articles that were submitted through the Manuscript Submission System became stalled in the deposit process when authors/investigators did not complete all of the required approvals.

After several years of discussions and experimentation with the deposit process, the mandatory policy took effect in April 2008. While the policy now required authors to submit their final manuscripts, there were no consequences or immediate repercussions for noncompliance.[9] Regardless, this radically changed compliance rates: The rate of submissions by authors and publishers more than doubled within four months of the policy becoming mandatory. In 2009, 70 percent of published articles declaring NIH funding were submitted to PMC. There was an increase in participating publishers; 40 percent of the submissions were deposited by the journal without intervention by the author.[10] Based on NIH data, by the end of 2008, compliance was reported as being 49 percent, in 2009 it rose to 70 percent, and by May 2012 it was 75 percent.[11] However, NIH, Congress, and the public expected higher compliance rates. While making the policy mandatory did result in more submissions, it was still a far cry from full compliance.

In late 2012, NIH announced increased enforcement with repercussions for noncompliance with the policy: "NIH informs grantees that in spring, 2013, at the earliest, NIH will delay processing of non-competing continuation grant awards if publications arising from that award are not in compliance with the NIH public access policy."[12] Given the five-year time span between implementing the mandatory policy in 2008 and enforcing it in 2013, many investigators had accumulated a long list of noncompliant articles. Investigators now needed to ensure that all of the articles they had published since April 2008 based on NIH-funded research were added to PMC in order to be in full compliance with the public access policy.

The literature contains examples of how other institutions developed methods and processes for supporting public access policy compliance.[13–17] Most of these reports predate the 2012 notice and do not specifically address managing compliance in the face of a possible loss of funding for noncompeting renewal grants. Here we describe how Duke University, and particularly the Medical Center Library and Archives, responded to the NIH public access policy. We focus on the decision points we faced that many other institutions may also encounter.

NIH-FUNDED RESEARCH PUBLICATIONS AT DUKE

Given Duke's strong record of biomedical publication output, the library had been keeping abreast of changes to the public access policy since 2005. As soon as drafts of the policy were released, we began alerting research deans, department chairs, administrative research offices, and faculty members to the possibility of changing requirements connected to NIH funding.

The public access policy is only one facet of a larger discussion about the need for researchers to acknowledge funding sources. At about the same time the initial policy was rolling out, DTMI and other research administrative offices began to more strongly promote the need for researchers to acknowledge federal funding— from NIH and other agencies—in manuscripts. Faculty awareness of the need to cite all funding sources was also heightened by increased pressure from the biomedical field and the general public for more transparency in identifying sources of support and potential conflicts of interest. Duke's 2013 CTSA renewal application also increased the focus on properly attributing publications to NIH-funded research and resources. DTMI staff members were assigned to track publications and to ensure that relevant grants were being acknowledged.

The library realized that this focus on citing grant numbers meant that more and more articles would be linked to NIH funding, both old and new, and we knew the scope of the problem would only grow. We had been using a Web of Science search to track Duke Medicine faculty publications for years. Our data showed that Duke authors have published four to five thousand biomedical articles each year since 2005. Based on the number of articles in the NIH Public Access Compliance Monitor we estimated that approximately one thousand to one thousand two hundred articles each year have been linked to NIH funding. As the policy changed from encouraged to mandatory with potential loss of funding, we became even more proactive in institutional compliance efforts and increased our efforts to work with DTMI and CRU administrators to ensure compliance steps were followed.

COMPLIANCE MANAGEMENT ROLE

When the public access policy became mandatory in 2008, the library reached out to the university research offices to discuss implications of the policy and institutional strategies. Meetings with the research deans and provosts, as well as other offices, revealed that while people had a vague knowledge of the policy, no one understood the full process for compliance. There was also confusion among authors and administrators since some manuscripts were submitted by publishers and others were not. The library volunteered to assist with communicating with researchers about the new mandatory policy and provided resources and training materials. Announcements went out to the faculty from the vice dean, and an institutional letter to publishers was developed explaining that Duke expected them to assist their authors with compliance. Web materials were posted, and numerous presentations were delivered to departments, centers, and grants administration offices. However, without specific repercussions or consequences for noncompliance, busy faculty members viewed this step of the research process as a low priority. The library continued to discuss this issue with research units, but since it was often difficult, if not impossible, to determine what was and was not compliant, our related services fell into a more reactive role, responding to specific questions as they arose.

When NIH published its 2012 notice that funding could be withheld for policy noncompliance, we recognized the urgent need to have another discussion with research offices about the potential impact of this change. After attending the NIH webcast "Changes to the NIH Public Access Policy and the Implications to Awards, NIH Grants, and Funding"[18] in January 2013, we identified potential roles for the library in the compliance process and opportunities for us to bring our expertise and experience to the work ahead.

We initiated a discussion about planning Duke's response to the policy changes with major stakeholders, including the Duke Office of Clinical Research, which provides navigation, tools, and training to support the conduct of clinical research,[4] and the Office of Research Administration (ORA), which provides technological tools, educational opportunities, and services for grants management.[19] Additionally, representatives from main campus were invited due to the number of NIH-funded researchers in other disciplines.

Prior to this meeting, we utilized the new Public Access Compliance Monitor (PACM), which provides access to compliance data, to analyze the extent of the issue. The initial report showed that Duke had more than 1,600 noncompliant articles since 2008. This involved the work of more than six hundred faculty members and represented a compliance rate at about the national average (74 percent). While some of the noncompliant articles did not fall under the policy due to acceptance dates or publication type, it was clear there was significant work to be done to bring Duke researchers into compliance.

During our meeting, we shared this data and reviewed the compliance process. We also discussed the various tools required for achieving and maintaining compliance. DOCR and ORA had the benefit of extensive knowledge of the grant process and experience using eRA Commons. However, they were not familiar with My NCBI and My Bibliography or the NIHMS. On the other hand, while the library had experience using My NCBI and knowledge of NIHMS, we had little experience with eRA Commons.

In addition to considering existing expertise, we also looked at how much time and manpower each group had available to devote to managing compliance. At the time of our initial meeting in early 2013, both of the research offices were very busy working on compliance with new ClinicalTrials.gov requirements. Additionally, DOCR was working to implement a new electronic health record system and to integrate this system into the clinical research environment. As a result of these ongoing projects, neither office had much manpower or resources to devote to public access policy compliance.

The Medical Center Library and Archives had both time and the staff expertise available to dedicate to the project. Therefore, it was decided that the library would lead the university's efforts to manage compliance, with support from DOCR and ORA. This has proved to work well over time. Although the library has managed most of the work, DOCR and ORA have both provided assistance when needed, particularly with troubleshooting problems and reaching out to researchers.

APPROACHING THE COMPLIANCE PROCESS

Designating the library to manage compliance was only the beginning; there was still a lot of work to do. In early 2013, only two members of the library staff understood the policy and the processes involved in compliance proficiently enough to teach others. The pending job was much larger than two people could handle; therefore, our first step was to recruit more librarians to participate. We assembled a team of people with a broad range of expertise and knowledge that would be particularly useful for this endeavor. The "NIH Library Team" included library liaisons to biomedical research, nursing, and medicine, as well as members of our collections and administrative departments.

After selecting our team we needed to train team members as quickly as possible; these group training sessions also provided an opportunity to test content and materials that would later be used to train investigators and research staff. Once everyone had a basic understanding of the policy and the compliance process, the team brainstormed how we could best approach the larger task of managing compliance.

We knew that there were many different strategies for managing compliance, including depositing on behalf of authors or providing instruction and support. In 2008, the library had offered to complete the NIHMS submission process for authors and created a system to collect manuscript files and all the associated information required by the manuscript submission system. The only two authors who tried the system reported that it was easier to submit directly, and the library shut down the system within the year. Our team decided not to resurrect this service given that authors would need to submit to us everything they would submit to NIHMS. Therefore, a submission service would not really save time; it would just add a middleman.

Once we decided not to mediate deposits, we began to tackle the issue of noncompliance. To start, we debated whom we should contact to resolve noncompliance for each article: the authors, the PI for the related grant, the publisher, or a combination of these. We decided to focus our initial efforts on contacting PIs for several reasons. First, we had too many articles that were noncompliant for contacting publishers to be a viable option. Even if publishers agreed to submit the articles, the authors would still need to approve the submissions in NIHMS to complete the deposit process. Additionally, contacting the authors proved complicated as the authors were often not affiliated with Duke, or had left Duke since publishing. Although we ran into similar issues with some PIs, the majority were either still affiliated with Duke or easier to find. Furthermore, as the PIs are ultimately responsible for ensuring that articles resulting from their grant funding are compliant, they have the most to lose if an article is not compliant, and thus the most motivation to fix noncompliant articles.

Notifying Principal Investigators

After we identified PIs as the initial point of contact for noncompliant articles, we discussed how to compile useful information to send them. We decided to create individualized reports for each PI including PACM data for publications for each PI-associated grant. We added color-coding and short descriptions of various compliance issues and collated articles with the same compliance issues to help investigators better understand what they needed to do to achieve compliance. We also investigated any article we thought might be exempt from the policy in order to provide better instructions for efficient handling of those articles. Over time, we had fewer noncompliant articles and fewer PIs to contact so we were able to increase the amount of detail and individual tailoring of reports to better assist researchers.

We then created e-mail templates to notify investigators of noncompliant articles. We discussed how to best formulate an e-mail that would both catch the attention of a busy PI and convey the necessary information. We opted for strong wording in both the title and opening sentences of the e-mail to convey a sense of importance and urgency, we included only brief instructions in the body of the e-mail, and we attached more detailed instructions. The attached instructions provided detailed help for compliance steps, such as setting up a My NCBI account. To reduce our workload and streamline communications, we created several different master documents, each with a combination of instructions for different noncompliance issues. This helped to generate tailored communications. For example, if a PI had several noncompliant articles and they all had the same issue (e.g., needed to be submitted to NIHMS), then we could easily send instructions to resolve only that specific issue. On the other hand, if a PI had several noncompliant articles with different issues (e.g., needed to be submitted to NIHMS; needed to be approved in NIHMS; needed their status changed in My Bibliography), then we could send a document with that combination of instructions.

Supporting the Research Community

While this was a great first step, sending e-mail notifications to PIs does not sufficiently address the problem of noncompliance. The process of determining if an article falls under the policy, determining how an article needs to be submitted, and completing the process of submitting an article is complicated, and there can be many challenges at many points along the way. Support can take many forms—in our case, we provided extensive in-person and online support.

Initially we created two separate, online detailed guides. We developed a general guide from one that was originally created in 2008 to describe the policy: http://guides.mclibrary.duke.edu/nihpublicaccess. The second guide focused more specifically with the steps involved in making articles compliant: http://guides.mclibrary.duke.edu/nihpapcompliance. Both guides contain screenshots and diagrams to illustrate the process of compliance and the steps involved. We provided links to relevant sections of the guide that were included in the standard e-mails we sent; the guides were also very useful for responding to e-mail questions.

In addition to developing and maintaining the online guides, we presented at numerous departmental meetings and large seminars, as well as hosting many workshops at the library. Through in-person instruction we reached 442 people between July 2012 and June 2014. Several sessions were live-streamed or recorded, one of which was uploaded to YouTube and linked to the library guide on our NIH Public Access Policy Compliance Guide (http://guides.mclibrary.duke.edu/nihpapcompliance).

After the first rounds of training were completed, the most used and most effective support we offered was individual consultations. We met with PIs and research staff in person or by phone and encouraged people to call, e-mail, or instant message us with questions. Between July 2012 and June 2014, we conducted 127 consultations with 160 people for a total of seventy-five hours. PIs and staff members who contacted us had a variety of questions. Initial questions focused on how to complete the basic steps and troubleshoot technical issues. Over time questions tended to focus more on dealing with problem issues, including logging in with expired passwords, articles not submitted by publishers in time, or claiming articles in NIHMS. After a year of sending personalized e-mails, additional strategies were utilized:

- Providing customized noncompliance reports for centers, grants with a multiple PIs, and departments;
- Identifying "high-risk" PIs, those with looming deadlines for research project progress reports (RPPR) for noncompeting renewals and sending them a special notice;
- Reaching out to PIs who left Duke and had easy-to-find contact information;
- Locating authors still at Duke who might be able to address problem citations;
- Sending separate reminders for manuscripts needing initial or final renewals;
- Requesting assistance from publishers for articles published before 2013, the most difficult ones for PIs and authors to handle;
- Working with main campus researchers directly and not through the main grants office;
- Providing main campus liaison librarians with reports of faculty out of compliance in their areas; and
- Communicating that compliance would be needed for future annual reports and possibly grant proposals.

Working closely with DOCR enhanced our communications strategy. We wrote articles for research newsletters that went out to research staff and faculty. Many of these articles also appeared in the library's blog and newsletter. Presentations were made at a "Research Wednesday" seminar where administrative and regulatory processes, tools, and resources are discussed by those managing research protocols. The content of the communications shifted over time from how to reactively handle outstanding manuscripts to how to proactively track and monitor publications.

Additionally, the library continued to work with and update the research offices on overall institutional compliance. Outstanding compliance issues were analyzed by the number of publications, PIs, and departments involved, and reports were sent to DOCR, ORA, the vice dean and provost for research, and other groups. The reports both celebrated the accomplishments as compliance rates rose and highlighted challenges when requests to address problems were ignored by faculty. These offices continued to provide guidance and feedback to the library team and were confident that the library could handle the work without additional oversight.

The library also met with research groups, such as DTMI and the Duke Clinical Research Institute (DCRI), to talk about how to proactively ensure compliance moving forward. In addition to citing directly funded projects, DTMI wanted investigators to cite Duke's CTSA grant whenever award-sponsored core resources were being used. The increased focus on citing grants resulted in discussions of complex issues. For example, how can PIs track publications that they didn't know about (e.g., papers authored by collaborators on which the PI is not an coauthor), or that may not have cited the grant? The library team recommended that PIs advise all collaborators to notify the PI of all pending journal articles. Additionally, we advised and assisted in saving searches in PubMed and other databases by grant numbers or authors' names for departments and centers whose large training or core grants often support numerous investigators.

We continue to identify new opportunities for library involvement in compliance management. For example, in 2015 NIH launched the new, required format for its Biosketch, investigator biographical information provided as part of the grant application. The announcement of a new Biosketch format raised concerns among researchers and their staff members, who in turn contacted librarians for advice. This created another opportunity for the library to highlight compliance issues and educate researchers. In response, the library scheduled a meeting with stakeholders from various research offices. During this meeting, we planned training sessions and identified ways to alert the research community to the new requirements, restate the importance and process for compliance, and encourage the use of SciENcv,[20] the new online system for generating Biosketches.

The new Biosketch gives researchers the opportunity to highlight their impact on science within the biography and to link to their full publications list in My NCBI.[21-22] While the new Biosketch does not require full compliance with the NIH public access policy, citations in the Biosketch are pulled from My Bibliography, which immediately alerts authors to compliance issues. As researchers will have to demonstrate compliance for future annual progress reports, this provides another opportunity for us to discuss the compliance process.

CHALLENGES

Every institution with NIH-funded research will have to deal with the issue of how to manage compliance with the NIH public access policy. The magnitude of the issue will vary greatly depending on the amount of funding and number of investigators and grants at that institution. The more funding, investigators, and grants at an institution, the more complicated managing compliance will be. A number of entities should be consulted in determining who and how compliance will be managed, including offices that oversee grant management, research offices, compliance offices, and the library. If possible, it is important to include from the beginning any stakeholder who might deal with helping investigators comply with the policy in order to open up communications between all parties. An institution's solution may be similar to ours at Duke, with one entity managing most of the work, or it may be more diffuse, with individuals from multiple entities working together. The important aspect is that all relevant parties should be in communication with each other.

An immediate challenge we needed to overcome was the inability to fully view and experience the entire compliance process. One librarian on our team had an eRA Commons account and could view the systems and process. Most of the members of our team did not have this level of access and often could not replicate a problem or process as they attempted to help a researcher. For example, one essential step in compliance management is linking a My NCBI account to the PIs' eRA Commons account. Librarians were unable to do this step because they didn't have an eRA Commons account and therefore weren't able to work through this part of the process themselves before assisting others. Additionally, librarians couldn't see the information available in a linked account and had to rely on screenshots or online instructions, which were minimal in early 2013. To overcome this challenge, the librarian with access to eRA Commons developed detailed online instructions with screenshots for team members and researchers to use. Similarly, in the first few months, team members relied heavily on the sole team member with PACM access to answer questions and help them "see" the system as they answered researchers' questions. Although it is nearly impossible to overcome this obstacle without becoming an NIH-funded researcher, having at least one team member with an eRA Commons account allows access to many of the functions of the systems. And fortunately, more documentation and resources are available today than there were in early 2013.

Dealing with noncompliance in the case of large, multisite grants or grants citing a NIH-funded core also proved daunting. Many authors and PIs forgot they were involved in older projects or did not know a manuscript had been submitted by authors at another site. In early 2013, the PACM system listed every PI associated with a grant even though often many of these PIs were not directly associated with particular projects or linked via a subaward. For example, Duke was awarded grants that provided research equipment or other resources that would be commonly shared by many researchers. The expectation was that anyone using these resources would cite that large resource grant. Compliance reports also included older grants that expired before 2008 but that were cited by authors in their acknowledgments. One extreme example that required countless communications and caused lots of confusion was an article that acknowledged forty separate grants from twenty institutions, including one resource grant that ended prior to 2008. As a result of this single publication, 121 Duke investigators were listed on the noncompliance report. These frequent discrepancies complicated communication in a number of ways, including identifying the appropriate PI to address the issue; trying to convince one PI to take responsibility; and dealing with confusion as to why a grant was cited. Fortunately, the NIH database was updated to remove many of these older grants, but even now data from pre-2008 funded studies are being analyzed in articles that acknowledge much older grants.

Finding correct e-mail addresses can be challenging even within a centralized directory system. The Duke system contains different formats of names, and these did not always match the NIH listing of the PI name. Because author names in the PACM spreadsheet did not match existing faculty lists, it was not feasible to use an automated process to do this work. We did obtain two spreadsheets that provided a listing of faculty names; this helped identify the current faculty. A spreadsheet from DOCR that provided faculty listings with research staff gave us another contact point. Sometimes PIs were not in the Duke central mail system and their current addresses had to be located. For those PIs who were no longer at Duke, librarians used their search skills to locate the researcher's current institutional home and e-mail address. For deceased PIs and for many who had retired, the hunt turned to authors of the article who might still be at Duke; we often contacted ORA to see if a Duke PI took over the grant. As we discovered discrepancies and uncovered current e-mails, we created a master reference list of problematic contacts to save time in future efforts.

We also experienced the problem of capturing the attention of researchers and sustaining their interest once we had their attention. We had to convey that the policy was now mandatory, with serious repercussions for noncompliance, at the same time that researchers and research managers were trying to deal with other compliance issues, including ClinicalTrials.gov registration and reporting. The numerous acronyms (My NCBI, My Bibliography, eRA Commons, RPPR, NIHMS, etc.) of the systems involved in compliance created a confusing alphabet soup. This new "foreign language" was difficult for librarians to explain and for researchers to grasp. There was already confusion among the article identification numbers involved in compliance, including PubMed ID (PMID) and PubMed Central ID (PMCID) for citations in those databases, and the number (NIH Manuscript Submission System ID [NIHMSID]) assigned to a manuscript in the compliance process. Finally, at Duke, we had another competing priority—a new faculty profiling system called Scholars@ Duke. This launched in May 2013, at the same time that compliance became a funding issue. The library made the decision not to promote Scholars@Duke until the compliance issues were addressed. While we were available to answer questions about this resource, our priority was working with faculty on the public access policy.

LESSONS LEARNED

Working with key research offices is essential. The offices need to understand the expertise that the library can bring to compliance and research issues and be comfortable in relying on them to provide services to the research community. It is also critical to have the support of these offices when problems occur or if researchers become angry or frustrated with processes. Administrative offices can wield more power over recalcitrant faculty and departments should this become necessary. In addition, there may be communication and training structures in place that you can leverage for your work. Ensuring that these partners are informed of the status of your work, challenges, and new ideas is an essential part of the ongoing partnership. One way to maintain an open channel of communication is to send out progress reports; this ensures everyone is informed and that your work remains highly visible.

For librarians supporting compliance with the NIH public access policy, one of the biggest challenges to overcome is gaining access to the Public Access Compliance Monitor. To fully understand and access details on compliance you need access to both eRA Commons and the PACM. Each institution will have a different method of managing accounts in eRA Commons, and institutions may be more or less restrictive in determining who can have access. Fortunately, prior to the introduction of the new requirements and PACM, one librarian had already successfully argued the usefulness of having access to eRA Commons and had established an account. Thus, when discussions of which group should manage compliance began, it was easier to suggest the library. For other libraries, we would encourage arguing for access to PACM if you plan to take on the primary role of managing compliance. If you are unable to gain an account, ensure that you have a close working relationship with those who do have access.

Obtaining and maintaining the attention of busy faculty and research staff can be difficult. Messages have to be repeated time and time again. Find different venues for getting your message or information to your target community. Use different approaches—e-mail, print, websites, and in-person sessions—each approach will appeal to different people. Try to find clever ways to get people's attention through special headlines or subject lines. Look for opportunities to be involved.

Timing is critical, and the library needs to be poised—and willing—to take advantage of unforeseen opportunities. Had we delayed in contacting research administrators, individuals less qualified than our librarians would likely have been assigned the task of addressing compliance issues. By being proactive and reaching out, even though we were not entirely sure of the time commitments and available resources, we became an essential element in the university process instead of a bystander trying to fit into someone else's system. This worked again with the Biosketch—another example of successful outreach to offices we knew might be struggling with the same questions rather than waiting for someone to create a solution that did not include us.

Learning from other librarians was very helpful. Other libraries have taken different approaches, and we have learned from them at conferences, through webinars, and through discussion lists. We have taken great ideas and applied them, as well as shared our own experiences.

Quickly identify what works well and abandon or change what does not. We have learned from our mistakes! Stern-sounding e-mails, complex instructions, and overwhelming spreadsheet reports did not work well and resulted in frustrated faculty and staff. We learned to simplify and tailor language and reports to gain cooperation and collaboration rather than resistance. We abandoned lengthy instruction sheets and started integrating briefer instructions into e-mails and reports. Training sessions for groups worked well in the beginning, but one-on-one sessions for PIs or staff members were clearly the better approach in our environment. Walk-in sessions and "clinics" for faculty became less necessary over time. We were flexible enough to abandon an approach and try other methods as needed.

OUTCOMES AND FUTURE PLANS

The most critical outcome to the university and researchers is our policy compliance rate. Our work with investigators has raised the compliance rate from 74 percent to 97 percent. Most researchers are now fully compliant, including those with older citations, which were the most difficult to resolve. Unlike the early months of 2013, researchers no longer run the immediate risk of having their funding withheld due to noncompliance. Senior researchers and their staff now refer new investigators to our librarians, resources, and services to help ensure compliance from the beginning. The university's research deans and officers have one less compliance concern, and the research community is more aware of the steps needed to stay in compliance.

We intend to continue our compliance work. To this end, we are building an internal database to support compliance management within our team. Currently, PACM reports are generated as .csv files and then saved as spreadsheets. While staff members have figured out clever ways to sort and reformat data in these spreadsheets, they are still difficult to use. To assist researchers, we have reviewed articles to see if they might be exempt (not peer-reviewed research), if grant information was wrong, or to identify coauthors who might be contacted in addition to the PI. This is all useful information to track in order to prevent duplication of work or provide guidance if similar issues arise in the future. The database we are developing will provide a way to collect this additional data so that it is easily shared among the team and to prevent us from duplicating effort. The database will also match the PMID against the PubMed record and download the full citation, which is often required when contacting publishers for assistance.

We would like to establish best practices and working guidelines for proactive tracking of publications, internal reporting among PIs, and subawards. The library has been providing individual consultations on how to identify new publications and track work by coinvestigators, but broader communications and educational materials are essential. In developing these assets we need to continue to work with research offices and ensure guidelines are integrated into their resources and training.

Duke University has an instance of VIVO called Scholars@Duke that creates and hosts profiles for faculty, including a list of their publications. A software program harvests the publication data from a number of databases, including PubMed, but not from My Bibliography. Ideally, integration between the systems would eliminate the current duplication of effort; as it stands, faculty must update publication lists both in Scholars@Duke (by acknowledging that they are the author) and for My Bibliography (by linking relevant PubMed citations to My Bibliography). It would streamline the process if publication data could be easily shared between the systems. We are working with the provost and other relevant offices that oversee this system as a future goal for Duke.

Finally, other government agencies are issuing public access policies similar to the NIH policy. The policies issued by the Agency for Healthcare Research and Quality (AHRQ)[23] and NASA[24] use the NIHMS system and PMC to submit and archive publications. Other agencies may take the same approach as they issue their policies. We expect there will be an increase in the number of publications that fall under public access policies and an increasing number of investigators who need to understand the systems and steps involved in achieving and maintaining compliance.

CONCLUSION

Taking on the role of managing compliance with the NIH public access policy has been both challenging and rewarding for our library. Although it has required a great deal of time, and often caused a great deal of frustration, it has also led to many benefits. The partnership among the library, DOCR, and ORA has strengthened, leading to additional collaborations. DOCR, ORA, and other offices now contact us more often than they did previously and look to us for support and input related not only to the policy but also to many other areas. Additionally, this work has increased the visibility of the library within our research community. We have helped numerous PIs and their research staff, who in turn now look to us for help with other needs; these PIs now view us as an important resource and source of support for their research.

We also have stronger relationships with our CTSA and within research centers, institutes, and multisite grants. While we do not receive funding from our CTSA, the library has established a critical role within the CTSA research structure. We have built relationships with CTSA staff and researchers through ensuring publications cite NIH funding and comply with the policy. We have also developed a strong partnership with DOCR, a key component within the CTSA organization. We have successfully assumed a leadership role for institutional compliance with one set of NIH funding requirements, ensuring ongoing funding and contributing to the success of grant renewals.

We are now regarded as a true partner in the research community; this has yielded invitations to participate in special events. For example, the librarians hosted a table at Duke's Clinical Research Day, an event that focuses on all the offices and services that support research activities and is heavily attended by research managers and coordinators as well as faculty. The library started working with another office on a series of research-related presentations called Research Wednesdays and has been invited to be a regular part of those presentations. Our compliance work has also led to involvement in discussions about data sharing and management, issues related to human subjects research and institutional review boards, and Biosketch training. Overall, our proactive stance and leadership in matters of public access policy compliance has led to many other opportunities to partner in key areas.

NOTES

1. National Science Foundation. Rankings by total R&D expenditure. http://ncsesdata.nsf.gov/profiles/site;jsessionid=519A925E61C6701A1CAB3D9DDC0EE0B8?method=rankingBySource&ds=herd. Accessed March 1, 2015.

2. National Institutes of Health. NIH awards by location and organization. http://www.report.nih.gov/award/index.cfm?ot=&fy=2014&state=&ic=&fm=&orgid=&distr=&rfa=&om=n&pid. Accessed March 1, 2015.

3. Duke Medicine. Facts and statistics. http://corporate.dukemedicine.org/AboutUs/Facts_and_Statistics. Accessed March 1, 2015.

4. Duke Office of Clinical Research, Duke University School of Medicine. What's new at DOCR? http://docr.som.duke.edu/. Accessed March 1, 2015.

5. Duke Office of Clinical Research, Duke University School of Medicine. Clinical research units. http://docr.som.duke.edu/clinical-research-units/cru-pages. Accessed March 1, 2015.

6. National Institutes of Health. NIH budget. http://www.nih.gov/about/budget.htm. Updated January 29, 2015. Accessed March 1, 2015.

7. National Institutes of Health. Analysis of comments and implementation of the NIH public access policy. September 30, 2008. http://publicaccess.nih.gov/analysis_of_comments_nih_public_access_policy.pdf. Updated October 3, 2008. Accessed March 1, 2015.

8. National Institutes of Health. Policy on enhancing public access to archive publications resulting from NIH-funded research: NOT-OD-05-022. February 3, 2005. http://grants.nih.gov/grants/guide/notice-files/NOT-OD-05-022.html. Accessed March 1, 2015.

9. National Institutes of Health. Revised policy on enhancing public access to archived publications resulting from NIH-funded research: NOT-OD-08-033. January 11, 2008. http://grants.nih.gov/grants/guide/notice-files/NOT-OD-08-033.html. Accessed March 1, 2015.

10. Lipman DJ. Public access to federally funded research: Testimony before the Committee on Oversight and Government Reform Subcommittee on Information Policy, Census and National Archives, United States House of Representatives. July 29, 2010. http://www.hhs.gov/asl/testify/2010/07/t20100729c.html. Updated June 13, 2013. Accessed February 18, 2015.

11. Poynder R. Open access mandates: Ensuring compliance. *Open and shut?* (blog). May 18, 2012. http://poynder.blogspot.com/2012/05/open-access-mandates-ensuring.html. Accessed March 1, 2015.

12. National Institutes of Health. Upcoming changes to public access policy reporting requirements and related NIH efforts to enhance compliance: NOT-OD-12-160. December 21, 2012. http://grants.nih.gov/grants/guide/notice-files/NOT-OD-12-160.html. Accessed March 1, 2015.

13. Stimson NF. National Institutes of Health public access policy assistance: One library's approach. *J Med Libr Assoc.* 2009;97(4):238–40. doi:10.3163/1536-5050.97.4.002.

14. Keener M, Sarli C. Public access policy support programs at libraries: A roadmap for success. *Coll Res Libr News.* 2010;71(10):539–42.

15. Rosenzweig M, Schnitzer AE, Song J, Martin S, Ottaviani J. National Institutes of Health public access policy and the University of Michigan Libraries' role in assisting with depositing to PubMed Central. *J Med Libr Assoc.* 2011;99(1):97–99. doi:10.3163/1536-5050.99.1.018.

16. Lapinski PS, Osterbur D, Parker J, McCray AT. Supporting public access to research results. *Coll Res Libr.* 2014;75(1):20–33. doi:10.5860/crl12-382.

17. Taylor A. Libraries take on policy: Support for open access and open data. *Against the Grain* (Charleston, S.C.). 2014 Apr 1;26(2):28, 30, 32.

18. NIH Grants and Funding. Changes to the NIH public access policy and the implications to awards, NIH grants, and funding (webinar). January 15, 2013. http://grants.nih.gov/grants/webinar_docs/webinar_20130115.htm. Updated February 15, 2013. Accessed March 10, 2015.

19. Duke Office of Research Administration, Duke University School of Medicine. Mission, vision, values. http://research.som.duke.edu/home/mission-vision-values. Accessed March 1, 2015.

20. National Center for Biotechnology Information, U.S. National Library of Medicine. SciENcv background. http://www.ncbi.nlm.nih.gov/sciencv/background. Accessed March 1, 2015.

21. National Institutes of Health. New biographical sketch format required for NIH and AHRQ grant applications submitted for due dates on or after January 25, 2015. NOT-OD-15-024. November 26, 2014. http://grants.nih.gov/grants/guide/notice-files/NOT-OD-15-024.html. Accessed March 1, 2015.

22. Update: New biographical sketch format required for NIH and AHRQ grant applications submitted for due dates on or after May 25, 2015: NOT-OD-15-032. December 5, 2014. http://grants.nih.gov/grants/guide/notice-files/NOT-OD-15-032.html. Accessed March 1, 2015.

23. Agency for Healthcare Research and Quality. Public access to federally funded research: Publications and data. February 9, 2015. http://www.ahrq.gov/funding/policies/publicaccess/index.html. Accessed March 9, 2015.

24. National Aeronautics and Space Administration. NASA plan: Increasing access to the results of scientific research—Digital scientific data and peer-reviewed publications. November 21, 2014. http://science.nasa.gov/media/medialibrary/2014/12/05/NASA_Plan_for_increasing_access_to_results_of_federally_funded_research.pdf. Released February 11, 2015. Accessed March 9, 2015.

13

Taking Flight to Disseminate Translational Research

A Partnership between the Umass Center for Clinical and Translational Science and the Library's Institutional Repository

Lisa A. Palmer and Sally A. Gore

ABSTRACT

The archive eScholarship@UMMS is the University of Massachusetts (Umass) Medical School's open-access digital archive of research and scholarship managed by the Lamar Soutter Library. The library began collaborating with the Umass Center for Clinical and Translational Science (U-MCCTS) in 2011. The archive eScholarship@UMMS facilitates knowledge and resource sharing of the U-MCCTS by collecting and organizing its research products, including research retreat posters and presentations, community-engagement symposia products, the U-MCCTS newsletter, the U-MCCTS seminar series, and publications that are the result of U-MCCTS-supported research. The archive provides long-term stable URLs for access to content, which are highly discoverable in Google and other search engines, maximizing readership and impact of U-MCCTS products. U-MCCTS administrators receive usage statistics for inclusion in grant progress and assessment reports to demonstrate this public impact. From July 2011 to mid-July 2015, 657 U-MCCTS products were downloaded 43,380 times. Further, eScholarship@UMMS not only facilitates discovery of U-MCCTS products but also provides long-term preservation of these products, ensuring their accessibility beyond the U-MCCTS grant cycle. This case study, which is relevant to the sharing and dissemination phase of translational research, will explore this partnership, which has been a win-win for both the library and the U-MCCTS.

GETTING READY TO BOARD

The University of Massachusetts Medical School (UMMS) was founded in the 1960s and graduated its first class of physicians in 1974. We are the only public medical school in the state, and while our students specialize in many areas, our chief purpose is to train primary-care doctors. Today, the medical school is home to three graduate schools: the medical school, the Graduate School of Biomedical Sciences, and the Graduate School of Nursing.

Over the past decade, UMMS has become a thriving biomedical research center. Expansions in facilities, research funding, and faculty make the university a leader among academic health sciences centers in the United States.[1] In 2006, professor Craig C. Mello shared the Nobel Prize in Medicine with his colleague, Andrew Fire of Stanford University, for their discovery of RNA interference. Gene function and expression, as well as gene development continue to be prominent areas of work for UMMS researchers.

In 2010, the U-MCCTS received a twenty-million-dollar Clinical and Translational Science Award (CTSA) from the National Institutes of Health (NIH).[2] The award encompasses research across all five UMass campuses, establishing the U-MCCTS at the medical school. This award, along with major backing from the Commonwealth's Life Sciences Initiative, allows UMMS to develop new curricula, programs, and partnerships that are transforming the way medicine is taught; medical research, carried out; and health care, provided.

Throughout the growth of our campus, the Lamar Soutter Library sits at the center of service, evolving like our larger institution to meet its changing needs. For years, our focus was on providing very traditional library services to the medical students, access to resources, and instruction in the same. As the university expanded and technology changed everyone's lives, the library looked to new and different ways to remain at the heart of the academic community.

One of the most effective means we found for reaching the research community was through the passage of the NIH public access policy in 2008. The requirement of NIH-funded researchers to deposit their publications into PubMed Central was the perfect opportunity for us to gain access to departments and groups that had eluded us in the past. Here was a topic that they needed to understand, and they looked to the library to explain it to them. Building a collaborative working relationship with our Office of Research Funding helped us to be seen as the point of contact for educational purposes while they addressed issues of compliance. It also ensured that the library remained free of any bad feelings and frustrations on behalf of the researchers that arose from the policy. We were there to help, not police.

Once we had our foot in the door, we were able to share with these same groups some of the other resources we had available for them, most notably our institutional repository (IR), eScholarship@UMMS.[3] The library had launched eScholarship@ UMMS in 2006 to showcase the medical school's achievements in research and scholarship. Institutional repositories help universities manage and disseminate digital materials created by their faculty, staff, students, and administrative units. These digital materials are typically organized into "collections" by department, research group, or program and are in a wide range of formats, including articles (including preprints and postprints), audio files, book chapters, conference posters and presentations, data sets, dissertations and theses, e-books, reports, and videos. The primary benefit of institutional repositories is that they raise the visibility and enhance the accessibility of digital content by providing free, unrestricted, online access to these publications. Collections in IRs serve as showcases to attract prospective students, researchers, and faculty to a university and can help institutional groups manage and track their publishing output.

By the time the U-MCCTS was created in 2010, eScholarship@UMMS was well established and flourishing, with more than a hundred collections. We picked departments strategically, focusing on established relationships and projects involving the IR that we thought would be particularly suited for a group. One of these groups turned out to be the U-MCCTS.

TAXIING TO THE RUNWAY

(Sally) In 2011, I took a continuing-education class offered at the Modern Language Association's (MLA) annual meeting held in Minneapolis. Taught by Cathy Sarli and Kristi Holmes from the Becker Medical Library at Washington University Medical School (St. Louis), "Forging a Path for Translational Science Support at Your Institution" was an interactive session that left me with a whole list of ideas for ways that we could partner with the U-MCCTS.

I came back from the conference and immediately made an appointment with the center's director of operations, Nate Hafer. I knew Nate from having helped him with things related to the public access policy, as well as some literature searching. Lisa and I met him and one of his staff members with our list of ideas in hand:

- Conference/symposia event organization. The IR includes functionality for organizing a conference and publishing its proceedings. The U-MCCTS was about to hold its first research retreat, and eScholarship@UMMS would be an ideal tool for archiving the presentations and posters and making them accessible, now and in the future.
- Collection of grant-supported publications. We proposed to set up an automated alert in PubMed to search for new publications supported by the U-MCCTS grant. This alert would help bring these publications together into a cohesive collection in the IR and keep the collection updated. An RSS feed of new publications would be available to embed on the U-MCCTS website if they wished to take advantage of that functionality.
- Project collections. Individual collections of publications could be established for specific projects funded by the U-MCCTS. These would be similar to col-

lections already in the IR, which showcased the publications of specific research laboratories at the medical school.

• Newsletter publishing platform. We proposed to use the IR as both a publishing platform and an archive for the center's monthly newsletter.

I also wanted to create educational materials and standards on topics related to properly citing U-MCCTS-funded articles, as well as the public access policy and the use of My NCBI. Tracking publications related to the U-MCCTS was difficult, and it seemed like an ideal place where we could help.

TAKING OFF

(Lisa) We were excited about this proposed endeavor with the U-MCCTS for a number of reasons. We already possessed the tool and expertise—a mature, successful institutional repository coordinated by an experienced repository manager—that we could leverage for this project. Existing IR collections could demonstrate our "proof of concept." We hoped to achieve the following goals:

• Dynamic new (and previously unpublished) content for the IR;
• Increased usage/downloads;
• Increased campus visibility and awareness of library services and expertise;
• Successful demonstration of IR utilization for grant support; and
• New partnership with the U-MCCTS.

We anticipated that our proposed collaboration would also be persuasive and attractive to the U-MCCTS. The library has an acknowledged reputation at the medical school for teamwork and responsiveness, which would certainly be helpful. In preparation for a meeting, we identified additional positive benefits and outcomes for the center:

• Library services provided at no cost to them, utilizing infrastructure already in place at the medical school;
• Visually appealing display that could be customized to match the look and feel of the U-MCCTS website;
• Immediate exposure of U-MCCTS-supported scholarship through Google, Google Scholar, and other search engines to maximize readership and impact, more than simply a bibliography of published work;
• Wide dissemination of U-MCCTS scholarly products, both peer-reviewed publications and gray literature;
• Monthly usage statistics as evidence of impact; and
• Ease of participation.

The outcomes of the June 2011 meeting were very positive. The U-MCCTS staff immediately responded to the idea of creating a conference proceedings collection in the IR for their recent research retreat, which had produced about a hundred posters and presentations. Lisa sent Hafer comprehensive follow-up information and provided wording about eScholarship@UMMS for an e-mail that he agreed to send to all participants requesting that they submit their abstract, poster, or presentation for inclusion in the collection. They were also very much in favor of creating a collection of grant-supported research publications. The timing was excellent; while some publications were in process, none had been published at that point in time.

The U-MCCTS was not quite prepared to support project collections or to migrate their newsletter to the IR platform but agreed to revisit these initiatives down the line. They welcomed the idea of working closely with Sally to develop and disseminate educational materials about the NIH public access policy for their members.

Our role was to manage the setup and maintenance of the collections in eScholarship@UMMS, including serving as the liaison to the repository vendor. Other library responsibilities included gathering the content, submitting it into the IR with accurate and complete metadata, addressing copyright concerns, and handling overall management of the project. The U-MCCTS, as the content provider, provided background information and publication lists, sent out the requests for participation to the faculty, and provided encouragement and promotion of the project.

We immediately began to collaborate with U-MCCTS administration to specify the information needed by our IR vendor to build and design a customized research retreat website in the repository. For branding purposes, it was important to make the collection within eScholarship@UMMS look as if it was an official part of the U-MCCTS website. After much discussion and multiple iterative mock-ups, the eScholarship@UMMS site for the UMass Center for Clinical and Translational Science Research Retreat launched in July 2011.

Additional U-MCCTS collections were brought online later that year and over the next few years. In September 2011, we launched a conference proceedings website for the annual symposium of their community engagement section, featuring posters, abstracts, and presentations from the event.

A collection of grant-supported research publications was established in May 2012. For this collection, we routinely harvest metadata from PubMed for publications that cite our U-MCCTS grant number and add records for these publications into eScholarship@UMMS. Our process includes determining which version of the paper we can archive in the IR. For articles that are clearly open access with a Creative Commons license, the full text of the published articles is uploaded into the IR. If an article's publisher permits self-archiving of preprints or postprints—many publishers allow this as demonstrated in the SHERPA/RoMEO database of publishers' policies on copyright and self-archiving managed by the University of Nottingham[4]—we can contact the authors to encourage them to provide us with that version for uploading. For articles where the publisher does not allow self-archiving, or where a preprint or postprint is not available at the time of harvesting, we provide a link to the publisher's website or to a PubMed Central version if available.

In November 2014, we rounded out the U-MCCTS community in the repository with archives for the center's monthly newsletter and presentations from its seminar series (figure 13.1).

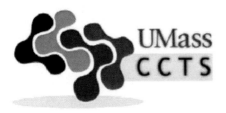

UNIVERSITY OF MASSACHUSETTS CENTER FOR CLINICAL AND TRANSLATIONAL SCIENCE

The goal of the University of Massachusetts Center for Clinical and Translational Science (UMCCTS) is to move laboratory discoveries into treatments for patients, to engage communities in clinical research, and to train a new generation of researchers. Through the center, we will facilitate greater efficiency and productivity of UMass investigators across campuses to enhance the public's health. The UMass Center for Clinical and Translational Science is part of a national Clinical and Translational Science Award (CTSA) consortium created to accelerate laboratory discoveries into treatments for patients. The CTSA program is led by the National Institutes of Health's National Center for Research Resources.

New! View current news stories and articles about UMCCTS research and news archives from 2014, 2013, 2012, and 2011.

Follow

Browse the *University of Massachusetts Center for Clinical and Translational Science* Collections:

Community Engagement and Research Symposium

UMass Center for Clinical and Translational Science Newsletter

UMass Center for Clinical and Translational Science Research Retreat

UMass Center for Clinical and Translational Science Seminar Series

UMCCTS Supported Publications

Figure 13.1. Screenshot of University of Massachusetts Center for Clinical and Translational Science collection page in eScholarship@UMMS, http://escholarship.umassmed.edu/umccts.

A LITTLE TURBULENCE

Although both the library and the U-MCCTS view our ongoing collaboration as very successful, the project has not been without its challenges.

Some researchers have been reluctant to deposit the full text of their research retreat posters into the IR because it is "work in process." They haven't finished working with the data, have goals of publishing it in the near future, feel their conclusions aren't fully formed, or do not want to publicly disclose on the Internet research that might lead to a patent. We've tried to overcome their hesitancy by providing embargo periods, and we've also compromised by accepting abstract-only submissions for posters. The U-MCCTS now includes language in their annual call for proposals that makes clear their expectation that posters and presentations will be archived in the IR, mentioning the benefits of doing so, such as permanent links, wide exposure, and usage statistics. The number of retreat submissions archived in eScholarship@UMMS has increased each year.

The other major challenge of this project has been limited library staff resources to populate the collections with content. Like many institutional repositories, we follow a mediated deposit model; library personnel deposit publications into the repository on behalf of faculty authors in order to reduce barriers to content recruitment. The U-MCCTS projects were particularly demanding because of the large number of original publications involved; for example, the 2014 research retreat produced 140 posters. Also, like many other institutional repositories, we have only one full-time employee dedicated to the repository (Lisa, who has additional duties but dedicates 50–75 percent of her time to the IR). Since we are a stand-alone graduate school, we can't draw from a pool of undergraduate work-study students. We have met the challenge for projects with large amounts of content as best we can by utilizing library assistants and library fellows to assist Lisa with high-priority projects and batch uploading content to the repository through spreadsheets.

One more minor challenge we experienced, which is common to any project involving websites, was keeping the design updated. The U-MCCTS redesigned their website and adopted a new logo in 2014. As a result, to maintain consistency, the library managed the process of making similar changes to the websites for the U-MCCTS collections in eScholarship@UMMS. This process was labor intensive but ultimately rewarding with the positive response of the U-MCCTS staff to the refreshed websites.

GLOBAL FLIGHT PATH

The potential benefits and outcomes we outlined for the U-MCCTS back in June 2011 have all come to fruition: wider dissemination and exposure of their research products through a collaboration that has not been burdensome to the center in terms of either cost or time. EScholarship@UMMS provides long-term stable

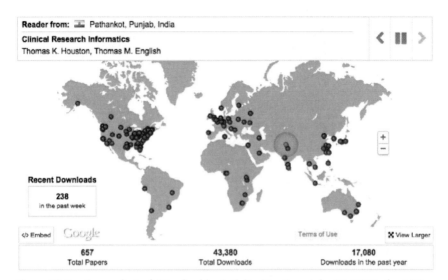

Figure 13.2. Screenshot of "Readership Activity Map" on July 17, 2015, for UMass Center for Clinical and Translational Science collection page in eScholarship@UMMS, http://escholarship.umassmed.edu/umccts.

URLs for access to their content, and these items are now highly discoverable in Google and other search engines; this maximizes readership and the overall impact of U-MCCTS products. Usage statistics are easily available for inclusion in grant progress and assessment reports to demonstrate this public impact. Between July 2011 and July 2015, 657 U-MCCTS publications were added to the repository and were downloaded a total of 43,380 times by readers all over the world (figure 13.2). Further, eScholarship@UMMS not only facilitates discovery of U-MCCTS products but also provides long-term preservation of these products, ensuring their accessibility beyond the U-MCCTS grant cycle. U-MCCTS director of operations Nate Hafer summarized his perspective as follows:

> One of the ways we measure impact is to track how UMass scholarship is disseminated out into the community. The eScholarship@UMMS repository is an excellent way we can showcase our work and follow usage metrics. It's exciting to see that our events from years past are still generating interest and contributing to the scientific process.[5]

We have also heard anecdotally from researchers that exposure to their research through eScholarship@UMMS has benefited them and their research. At the U-MCCTS research retreat in 2011, Barbara Olendzki, assistant professor of medicine, and her colleagues presented their poster entitled "Pilot Testing a Novel Treatment for Inflammatory Bowel Disease."[6] This poster quickly became one of the most downloaded items in eScholarship@UMMS, to the delight of Olendzki.

> We are really happy about this, and humbled by the response. Due in part to the call to action by the public with Inflammatory Bowel Disease (IBD), we have begun an

(underfunded) trial in patients with Crohn's Disease, and invite all patients with IBD to participate alongside those patients, to learn the IBD-AID diet. Without the tremendous response of our tiny pilot study, we would not have undertaken such a risk in forging forward with our current study. We greatly appreciate the exposure eScholarship@UMMS has provided for us in pursuing this groundbreaking and important research.[5]

Her coauthor David Cave, professor of medicine, was also pleased at the level of interest generated by the study's exposure through the institutional repository.

Diet and inflammatory bowel disease has become a hot area for public research as it relates closely to the intestinal microbiome, which in turn has been shown to influence disease activity of both Crohn's disease and ulcerative colitis. The astonishing level of interest, as measured by eScholarship@UMMS, in an abstract presented at a small meeting is a testament to this. Assessment of the benefit of dietary modification has been highly controversial, at least in part because it is difficult to measure benefit, and difficult for patients to be consistent in what they eat. Our preliminary data supports the benefit of the IBD-AID diet, in that some patients were able to reduce or eliminate the traditional medications used for IBD. We are now embarking on a randomized trial to try to provide conventional scientific evidence for the benefit of the diet. This type of trial is essential but a real challenge to execute with minimal funding.[5]

The benefits to the library have exceeded our expectations. We have added local, unique, digital collections to our institutional repository, increasing the value and novelty of our holdings. We now have a convincing narrative about the U-MCCTS and eScholarship@UMMS that we can share with researchers, administrators, and other librarians as we pursue additional collections of value.

FUTURE ITINERARIES

(Sally) Several years after that successful June meeting, the library's connection with the U-MCCTS is stronger than ever. I'm now a full-time member of the U-MCCTS staff, moving here in December 2014 to become their research evaluation analyst.

I was able to convince the U-MCCTS leadership of my skills and abilities for this position, in large part, because of many of the areas the library had moved or was moving and my role in those moves. The means and tools to measure scholarly communications and research impact are changing rapidly and, like the NIH public access policy, this is an area where our department took the lead in investigating trends, trying out tools, helping the library's administration persuade the university administration of the need for allocating resources to these tools (e.g., Scopus, SciVal, Plum Analytics), raising awareness of alternative metrics, and educating the research community on them. I'd had success in doing this within the community engagement section of the U-MCCTS; I'd presented a poster on the topic at the U-MCCTS research retreat; and all of the success we enjoyed with our partnership with the U-MCCTS gave me a personal vote of confidence from the leadership team. We work well together.

I came on board as the grant application for receiving another CTSA from NIH was just about due. Everyone was frantically writing and proposing and discussing how the different research cores and programs could grow in another funding cycle. I was there to write how we will evaluate these cores and overall program, and the one paragraph that was the easiest to write was the one describing how the U-MCCTS has and will continue to partner with the library to achieve some of our goals. From my new position, I was able to include items in our proposal that involve partnerships with the library in areas of instruction regarding alternative metrics, dissemination of information through the institutional repository, and continuing support in helping the U-MCCTS measure the impact of the scientific research generated by the center.

(Lisa) I continue to work closely with the U-MCCTS staff to ensure that the collections in the IR remain current, that the products are disseminated widely, and that metrics are kept to show the impact and reach of the center's work. Currently, Sally and her colleagues are planning to redesign their website, and I have suggested embedding the eScholarship@UMMS readership map or an RSS feed of recent publications to add dynamic content to their website. In the future I would also like to explore incorporating alternative metrics into the display of the U-MCCTS materials in eScholarship@UMMS.

My department in the library is involved in efforts to coordinate institutional support for research data management on our campus. Our main focus is on education and outreach, and the U-MCCTS would be a natural partner in these endeavors. We are also offering eScholarship@UMMS as a solution for publicly sharing research data, which may be useful to U-MCCTS investigators. The library has been a strong and valuable partner to the U-MCCTS, and I look forward to providing additional service in the future.

FLIGHT SOUVENIRS

Leverage What You Have. There are several natural connections between what librarians do and what CTSA centers on campuses need. We are the best resource for expertise and support when it comes to all things related to scholarly communications. Teaching, supporting, and promoting the NIH public access policy and open-access initiatives are perfect fits. These movements are leading to many opportunities to support work related to research dissemination, tracking research impact, and research evaluation. Depending upon one's skills, interests, and available resources, these are emerging as important possible roles for librarians and libraries. All are enhanced by IRs, and the library with a thriving IR is well positioned to build successful collaborations with their CTSA centers.

Put in the Time. Successful collaborations do not happen overnight. Building relationships is an essential part of the process and one that takes time. Going to programs sponsored by your CTSA, showing interest and support, and learning who's who and what's what are all important parts of the process. It's much easier to propose ideas to people that you know. It's also much more likely that you'll propose successful ideas if you have a good understanding of what your center does and how your library can best help.

Pretend That Everything Is a Pilot Project. Pilot projects are an opportunity to learn, be creative, expand the scope of your IR, work through technical and process issues, and produce a proof of concept to demonstrate your success. Welcome these opportunities.

Work with Other Academic Health Sciences Libraries. Our professional associations offer us a tremendous opportunity to network, learn, and share. Collaborations between CTSA centers are being highlighted at the national level now. If it's easier to approach a library colleague to propose an idea than your own CTSA office, give that a try. Working together is a huge part of translational science.

Don't Forget Your Institutional Repository. Institutional repositories provide new ways of engaging with researchers and can be a strong component of library services offered to your CTSA. Increased dissemination, exposure, and impact of their research products motivate faculty, departments, and CTSA centers. Supporting grants in this way to help researchers demonstrate the impact of publicly funded projects is an excellent utilization of the institutional repository.

NOTES

1. University of Massachusetts–Worcester. *US News and World Report.* 2015. http://grad-schools.usnews.rankingsandreviews.com/best-graduate-schools/top-medical-schools/university-of-massachusetts-worcester-04049. Accessed March 20, 2015.

2. UMass Center for Clinical and Translational Science. CCTS—UMass Medical School–Worcester. http://www.umassmed.edu/CCTS. Accessed March 15, 2015.

3. EScholarship@UMMS. EScholarship@UMMS at the University of Massachusetts Medical School. http://escholarship.umassmed.edu/. Accessed March 15, 2015.

4. SHERPA/RoMEO. University of Nottingham. http://www.sherpa.ac.uk/romeo. Accessed July 17, 2015.

5. EScholarship@UMMS reaches 1/2 million downloads (press release). Worcester, MA: Lamar Soutter Library; October 30, 2013.

6. Olendzki B, Persuitte G, Silverstein T, Baldwin K, Cave D, Zawacki J, Bhattacharya K, Ma Y. Pilot testing a novel treatment for inflammatory bowel disease. Poster presented at 2nd Annual UMass Clinical and Translational Science Research Retreat, May 2011; Shrewsbury, MA. http://escholarship.umassmed.edu/cts_retreat/2011/posters/15. Accessed March 15, 2015.

14

Capitalizing on Serendipity

Parlaying a Citation Report into a Publishing and Evaluation Support Program

Cathy C. Sarli, Kristi L. Holmes, and Amy M. Suiter

INTRODUCTION

Opportunities for medical libraries to engage in translational medicine activities can be found within existing library services and from the most ordinary of circumstances. The growing emphasis to demonstrate meaningful health outcomes resulting from translational medicine represents prime opportunities for medical libraries. Medical libraries have expertise in knowledge management and bibliometrics and are familiar with scientific research and publication practices. Building upon this foundation to provide solutions that help to illustrate meaningful health outcomes and translational efforts are among the services that medical libraries can offer in support of translational medicine activities on their campus.

This chapter reviews how a citation report request led to a retrospective analysis project to provide an investigator with a more robust narrative of impact resulting from a clinical trial research study. We describe the retrospective analysis project, highlight select project findings, and discuss the creation of a new service model at Bernard Becker Medical Library. Recent trends in the United States related to research impact are also reviewed. We hope this chapter will help inspire other medical libraries to parlay their expertise into programs that provide support for reporting of research impact for authors, investigators, research teams, and administrators.

THE RETROSPECTIVE ANALYSIS PROJECT: GENESIS

The date was May 17, 2007, and one of us had been recently assigned as a liaison librarian to the Department of Ophthalmology and Visual Sciences at Washington University School of Medicine in St. Louis.[1] I recognized a patron at Bernard Becker Medical Library as Mae O. Gordon, a faculty member from the department and director of the Vision Research Coordinating Center for the Ocular Hypertension Treatment Study (OHTS). I introduced myself to the patron and began to chat about library-related topics. One topic in particular was citation analysis. Gordon recalled seeing a poster about bibliometrics presented by Pam Sieving, informationist from the National Institutes of Health (NIH) Library (now retired), at the Association for Research in Vision and Ophthalmology's 2007 annual meeting.[2] Gordon wanted to know if it was possible to provide a citation report based on publications from a clinical research study.

The Ocular Hypertension Treatment Study was a randomized, controlled, multicenter clinical trial, 1992–2012, conducted in twenty-two clinical centers in the United States and funded by the National Eye Institute of the NIH (EY09307). OHTS was designed to determine whether lowering intraocular pressure (IOP) in individuals with ocular hypertension either delays or prevents the development of primary open-angle glaucoma (POAG). OHTS was the first trial to demonstrate definitively that treatment of elevated IOP delays or prevents the onset of glaucomatous damage. OHTS also identified risk factors for developing POAG, including older age, higher IOP, and larger cup/disc ratio, and was the first study to identify central corneal thickness (CCT) as an independent risk factor for the development of POAG.

THE CITATION REPORT

The first step was to identify the peer-reviewed journal articles generated by the OHTS investigators. A website for OHTS contained a bibliography of the publications and abstracts. Twenty-six peer-reviewed journal articles were identified from the OHTS bibliography.

The databases Scopus (Elsevier) and Web of Science (Thomson Reuters) were searched to locate citation data. From preliminary review, several of the OHTS journal articles were found to have high citation counts. Through the use of Thomson Reuters's Essential Science Indicators (ESI), it was determined that the citation counts from Web of Science exceeded the average citation rates and ranked high in the percentiles for the field of clinical medicine as well as for all fields covered by ESI. These findings were summarized in a report and delivered to Gordon.

The questions posed by Gordon were insightful and fundamentally challenged Becker Library to think about publication practices, citations, and ultimately research impact in a new way:

- Why did some articles garner high citation counts and others did not?
- Are citations indicative of significance?
- Do citations serve as a proxy for impact?
- What is a high-impact study?
- How could OHTS increase the likelihood of their research being translated into clinical applications?

While publications and citations were neatly quantifiable metrics, the report did not answer Gordon's questions as to significance and impact. Regular meetings were held throughout summer of 2007 to discuss the questions posed by Gordon.

THE INFLECTION POINT

Review of the literature to shed light on Gordon's questions revealed one publication of particular interest. A commentary by Wells and Whitworth outlined several examples of meaningful health outcomes and stated, "Traditional academic metrics of research output through peer-reviewed publications and citations are insufficient to satisfy society's expectation that public investment in research results in real benefit to the society."[3] Gordon's questions and this commentary underscored the necessity to continue the project as a retrospective analysis to locate evidence of meaningful health and societal benefits resulting from OHTS research study findings.

This impetus was an inflection point for the retrospective analysis project and subsequently led to the evaluation and impact program at Becker Library. A citation report is the initial step of any project or consultation involving assessment of research productivity or impact.

THE RETROSPECTIVE ANALYSIS PROJECT: CHALLENGES

The challenges were to further review the citing publications (e.g., why so many publications were citing the OHTS articles) as well as determine appropriate and credible secondary sources to find the answers to Gordon's questions. Before moving forward with the next phase of the retrospective analysis project, additional familiarity with the subject matter was required.

Reference materials, book chapters, and dissertations were reviewed to gain an understanding of glaucoma, the scientific progress advancements related to glaucoma, the vernacular, and the current knowledge base. The Computer Retrieval of Information on Scientific Projects (CRISP) database (now RePORTER, http://projectreporter.nih.gov/) was reviewed to find NIH-funded studies related to glaucoma. Trade publications and professional organizations and societies related to ophthalmology and glaucoma were also consulted (textbox 14.1).

TEXTBOX 14.1
Finding the Evidence

- Gain knowledge about the topic of the research study. Become familiar with acronyms, terminology, vernacular, standards, procedures, and so forth, related to the research topic.
- Read citing documents to determine why a publication was cited. Document the insights gained from review of the citing documents.
- Review the websites of organizations (professional/societal and governmental) and funding organizations related to the research topic.
- Use of nonbibliographic resources is required.
- Trade publications and gray literature are significant sources of evidence and clues.
- Anecdotal knowledge from investigators is required to identify clues of impact and to substantiate correlations from their research study to impact indicators.
- Be prepared for an iterative and messy process.
- Knowledge of the scientific research process in general is helpful as well as an understanding of publication patterns for the research topic and field.

Each publication that cited the OHTS articles was reviewed to learn why the OHTS articles were being cited as a means of contextualizing the citations. Next, the gray literature and other sources such as news media, popular press, government documents, technical reports, and policy statements were reviewed to find evidence of uptake of OHTS research study findings beyond citations. Search engines were used for locating gray literature and other sources not typically indexed by bibliographic databases. LexisNexis, ProQuest, and OCLC databases were used for locating popular press and related news media. The search terms used included:

- Names of the principal investigators: Michael Kass and Mae Gordon;
- Full name of the study: Ocular Hypertension Treatment Study;
- Acronym of the study name: OHTS; and
- Medical terms and acronyms related to OHTS: ocular hypertension, glaucoma, primary open-angle glaucoma (POAG), POAG suspect, central corneal thickness (CCT), intraocular pressure (IOP), pachymetry, and pachymeter (pachymetry is a technique used to measure CCT and is performed by a medical device called a pachymeter using ultrasound or optical methods).

A list of impact indicators was kept for reference over the course of the project. Impact indicators are defined as specific, concrete examples that demonstrate research impact as a result of a research finding or output. During the project, a number of indicators of impact were identified, beyond those related to OHTS.

THE RETROSPECTIVE ANALYSIS PROJECT: FINDINGS

A follow-up report was delivered to Gordon in September 2007 and noted specific impact indicators resulting from OHTS research study findings to answer the question of a high-impact study (textbox 14.2).

TEXTBOX 14.2
Examples of Impact Indicators for OHTS

Examples of impact based on citation data include the following:

- Citation rates for publications from the study exceed the median/average rates for that given field.
- Publications from the study are among the most frequently cited articles in journals for that given field.
- Publications from the study are cited in reviews, consensus developments, curriculum materials, continuing education materials, and insurance coverage positions.
- Publications from the study are cited in special articles devoted to highlights of discoveries/advancements in that particular field.

Examples of impact resulting from OHTS research study findings are as follows:

- Clinically effective approach in the management of a disease, disorder, or condition;
- Clinical guidelines;
- New "standard of care" for a disease, disorder, or condition;
- Identification of risk-assessment factors for a disease, disorder, or condition;
- Diagnostic criteria for a disease, disorder, or condition;
- Change in clinical practice;
- Procedure that is widely performed with demonstrated clinical efficacy;
- Cost-effective means for management of a disease;
- Measurement instruments;
- Increased quality of life for patients;
- Disease-prevention measures;
- Equipment or tool; and
- Current Procedural Terminology (CPT) codes.

A discussion of three examples of impact indicators resulting from OHTS research study findings follows below:

1. Clinical Guidelines

Clinical guidelines may be developed by government agencies, institutions, organizations such as professional societies or governing boards, or by the convening of expert panels and usually cite references from a research study whose findings were used to support the recommendations as noted in the guideline. Websites of professional organizations related to ophthalmology were searched as was the National Guidelines Clearinghouse (NGC) to locate clinical guidelines, if any (see figures 14.1 and 14.2).[4] Examples of clinical or practice guidelines that cited OHTS findings (as of 2007) included the following:

American Academy of Ophthalmology

- Primary Open-Angle Glaucoma Suspect Preferred Practice Pattern Guideline, 2005. (Available in eight other languages besides English)
- Primary Open-Angle Glaucoma Preferred Practice Pattern Guideline, 2005. (Available in eight other languages besides English)

American Optometric Association

- Quick Reference Guide for Clinicians Care of the Patient with Open-Angle Glaucoma, 2002.
- Optometric Clinical Practice Guideline on Care of the Patient with Open-Angle Glaucoma, 2002.

International Council of Ophthalmology / International Federation of Ophthalmological Societies

- Primary Open-Angle Glaucoma (Initial Evaluation), 2007.
- Primary Open-Angle Glaucoma (Follow-up Evaluation), 2007.
- Primary Open-Angle Glaucoma Suspect (Initial and Follow-up Evaluation), 2007.

2. American Medical Association Current Procedural Terminology (CPT) Codes

Current Procedural Terminology codes are published by the American Medical Association (AMA) and updated/revised annually.[5] The purpose of the CPT coding system is to provide uniform language that accurately describes medical, surgical, and diagnostic services. Adding, modifying, or deleting of CPT codes is performed by a review process involving a CPT editorial panel and a CPT advisory panel. Each proposed coding change must be supported by peer-reviewed literature. There are three categories of CPT codes:

Category I

Category I codes are the five-digit numeric codes included in the main body of CPT. These codes represent procedures that are consistent with contemporary medical practice and are widely performed.

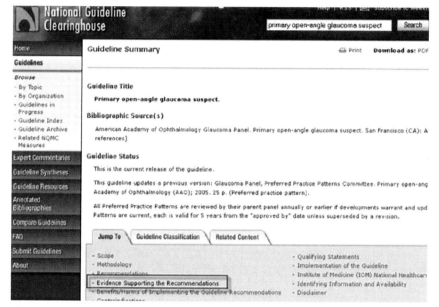

Figure 14.1. National Guidelines Clearinghouse (NGC) database record for a guideline summary that cites OHTS publications as "Evidence Supporting the Recommendations." The query used was "primary open-angle glaucoma suspect."

Foster PJ, Devereux JG, Alsbirk PH, Lee PS, Uranchimeg D, Machin D, Johnson GJ, Baasanhu J. Detection of gonioscopically occludable angles and primary angle closure glaucoma by estimation of limbal chamber depth in Asians: modified grading scheme. Br J Ophthalmol 2000 Feb;84(2):186-92. PubMed

Gordon MO, Beiser JA, Brandt JD, Heuer DK, Higginbotham EJ, Johnson CA, Keltner JL, Miller JP, Parrish RK 2nd, Wilson MR, Kass MA. The Ocular Hypertension Treatment Study: baseline factors that predict the onset of primary open-angle glaucoma. Arch Ophthalmol 2002 Jun;120(6):714-20; discussion 829-30. PubMed

Gutierrez P, Wilson MR, Johnson C, Gordon M, Cioffi GA, Ritch R, Sherwood M, Meng K, Mangione CM. Influence of glaucomatous visual field loss on health-related quality of life. Arch Ophthalmol 1997 Jun;115(6):777-84. PubMed

Kass MA, Heuer DK, Higginbotham EJ, Johnson CA, Keltner JL, Miller JP, Parrish RK 2nd, Wilson MR, Gordon MO. The Ocular Hypertension Treatment Study: a randomized trial determines that topical ocular hypotensive medication delays or prevents the onset of primary open-angle glaucoma. Arch Ophthalmol 2002 Jun;120(6):701-13; discussion 829-30. PubMed

Keltner JL, Johnson CA, Quigg JM, Cello KE, Kass MA, Gordon MO. Confirmation of visual field abnormalities in the Ocular Hypertension Treatment Study. Ocular Hypertension Treatment Study Group. Arch Ophthalmol 2000 Sep;118(9):1187-94. PubMed

Figure 14.2. National Guidelines Clearinghouse (NGC) database record that displays three OHTS publications in the "Evidence Supporting the Recommendations" section of the guideline summary.

Category II

Category II codes are supplemental tracking codes that are intended to be used for performance measurement. In compliance with ongoing changes being made because of Health Insurance Portability and Accountability Act (HIPAA) regulations, these codes provide a method for reporting performance measures.

Category III

Category III codes represent temporary codes for new and emerging technologies. They have been created to allow for data collection and utilization tracking for new procedures or services. To be eligible for a category III code, the procedure or service must be involved in ongoing or planned research. The rationale behind these codes is to help researchers track emerging technology and services to substantiate wide-spread usage and clinical efficacy.

Prior to 2002, a CPT code specific to pachymetry did not exist. Pachymetry was assigned as a category III code (CPT 0025T, Determination of corneal thickness, with interpretation and report, bilateral), effective January 2002. As of January 2004, a category I code (CPT 76514, Ophthalmic ultrasound, echography, diagnostic; corneal pachymetry, unilateral or bilateral, determination of corneal thickness) was assigned. The move from a category III to a category I was evidence that pachymetry, a "new and emerging technology," demonstrated clinical efficacy.

A clue as to a CPT code resulting from OHTS findings was found in a trade publication related to ophthalmology.[6] However, supporting documentation for implementation of new CPT codes related to pachymetry was not publicly available. Consultation with policy makers, with the help of Gordon, confirmed that the OHTS research study findings, along with other glaucoma research studies, resulted in the creation of a new CPT code, category III for corneal pachymetry in 2002, with follow-up to a CPT category I code in 2004.

3. Change in Clinical Practice

Discovery of a change in clinical practice was more elusive. This indicator required self-reported qualitative data from health-care providers. However, survey data provided important links between OHTS research study findings and changes in clinical practice. A survey of optometrists was referred to in a trade publication, and the source of the data was provided by the members of the Association of Vision Science Librarians (AVSL). Respondents to a 2003 survey of optometrists delivered through the national panel of Doctors of Optometry reported that the OHTS findings changed the way they manage glaucoma patients.[7]

THE RETROSPECTIVE ANALYSIS PROJECT: RECAP

A traditional citation report was not sufficiently robust to adequately describe the impact of OHTS research study findings and their resulting synthesis into meaningful health and societal outcomes such as new understanding of a disease, change in clinical practice, quality-of-life benefits, reduction in incidence of disease, and new research directions, to name a few. The OHTS publications that garnered high citation counts were those that described significant research findings. While citation data from these publications provided useful clues for further investigation, the citation counts themselves were not predictive of specific health outcomes.

The most difficult part of the retrospective analysis project was the lack of guidelines or recommended practices for locating evidence of impact indicators beyond bibliometric-based indicators. As noted in the 2010 *Journal of the Medical Library Association* article describing the methodology of the project, the process was neither tidy nor linear.[8] It was an iterative search process with various keywords and phrases used for queries. Reproducibility of queries, transience and diversity of sources, and lack of standard keywords were issues with this project as well as for all impact-analysis projects done since 2007 (textbox 14.3). The gray literature was very useful in locating specific indicators of impact as well as serving as clues for other indicators. Despite its drawbacks, the gray literature (trade publications in particular) contained documented sources to confirm a connection or link between an impact indicator and OHTS research study findings. The 2015 Sibbald work aptly describes both the challenges and the paybacks with gray literature for impact purposes.[9] In some instances, documentation as to a connection or link between a specific impact indicator and OHTS research study findings was not publicly available in the literature or other sources. For these instances, verbal and e-mail confirmation with appropriate parties was required to confirm a connection between specific impact indicators and OHTS.

TEXTBOX 14.3
Issues with Impact Analysis

- It is not a linear process, causing frustration at times.
- There is no automated means of locating evidence of impact.
- There is a lack of universal definitions for impact indicators.
- There is a time lag between research discovery and health and societal outcomes.
- The optimal time frame for starting an assessment of a research study is unknown.
- Supporting documentation for a specific impact indicator and a research study may not be publicly available.
- It may be difficult to establish a direct connection or link from a specific impact indicator and a research study.

The retrospective analysis project was not conducted in a vacuum. Sieving provided much support and encouragement as did the members of the AVSL who pointed out the availability of annual survey data from health-care providers in the field of ophthalmology. The survey data was a critical piece of evidence of impact as it indicated how the provision of health care had changed as a result of OHTS research study findings. Policy makers in the field also answered questions and referred to other sources of information for further investigation. In addition, Gordon was an essential partner (and continues to be) to the progress of the project.

THE RETROSPECTIVE ANALYSIS PROJECT: PRESENT DAY

As of this writing (May 2015), fifty-one peer-reviewed journal articles have been authored by the OHTS. A full list of publications and abstracts is available from the OHTS bibliography.[10] Becker Library continues to track OHTS. Some examples of impact indicators identified since 2007 include:

- Mobile application;
- New funded research studies expanding upon OHTS research study findings;
- New research direction in basic science research*;
- Increased usage of a term (CCT) related to OHTS in the literature;
- Cited in textbooks;
- Advanced careers of early stage investigators*; and
- Sixteen authorized requests for use of OHTS data in genotypes and phenotypes (dbGaP) database.[11]

In particular, two of the above examples (noted with an asterisk) were identified while discussing the project with Gordon. Consultation with Gordon revealed that some of the early-stage investigators who were involved with OHTS research findings were subsequently awarded independent R01 NIH awards that represent significant and innovative projects. Gordon and the other OHTS investigators also revealed that the OHTS research study findings spurred a new research direction in basic science research pertaining to the biomechanical properties of the eye. Genetic research is ongoing to determine if CCT is subject to heritability.

The two examples illustrate the importance of a team-based approach (library and research investigators) to identify and locate evidence of impact resulting from research findings. The process is iterative and requires ongoing consultation with investigators to discover anecdotal clues that may be revealed as indicators of impact and to confirm a connection between specific indicators and research study findings.

REVIEW OF PUBLICATION PRACTICES

One of the seminal questions posed by Gordon in 2007 focused on how OHTS could increase the likelihood of their research being translated into clinical applications. As part of this project, biomedical and general publication practices, including those by OHTS investigators, were reviewed to determine what factors, if any, enhance the discovery and uptake of published research findings. A number of practices were identified, and these helped to strengthen the outreach efforts of a newly

```
CN  - Ocular Hypertension Treatment Study (OHTS) Group
```

Figure 14.3.   MEDLINE/PubMed database record for an OHTS publication in the MED-LINE record view.

established scholarly communications program at Becker Library to promote strategies for authors to use to enhance the discovery and dissemination of their research.

One practice in particular that helped with discovery of impact indicators was that the OHTS investigators added the name of the study as a corporate author on their publications. This practice facilitates discovery of works by the OHTS investigators and serves as a branding function for the research study. As an example, the name of the study and the acronym are noted in the MEDLINE record display for an OHTS publication as a corporate author (see figure 14.3). More information on corporate authorship in MEDLINE/PubMed can be found in the Authorship in MEDLINE fact sheet.[12]

Another practice noted as being helpful for facilitating discovery and dissemination of OHTS research findings is the OHTS website, which includes the bibliography of publications and abstracts (http://ohts.wustl.edu/). Journal articles include the PMID (PubMed identifier) and are linked to the record in the MEDLINE/PubMed database. Conference presentations link to meeting abstracts and files presented at the meetings. At the time of the project, compliance with the NIH public access policy was only "highly encouraged" (not required until 2008), and most of the works were not available in PubMed Central (PMC). One recommendation made to OHTS was to deposit a copy of their journal articles into PMC. Toward this end, Becker Library contacted the publishers of the works to obtain permission to deposit a copy (final published version or final peer-reviewed version depending on publisher policies) of the journal articles in PMC.

THE RIPPLE EFFECTS

Assessing the Impact of Research Website

As a result of the project, a number of impact indicators related to bench and clinical research were identified including those not specific to the OHTS project. This list served as a checklist during the retrospective analysis project as a means of keeping track of what was located, documented, and not available. Indicators are defined as specific, concrete examples that demonstrate research impact. Examples of tangible impact indicators include research studies, clinical guidelines, legislation or policy, and quality-of-life metrics, among many others. The impact indicators were grouped under pathways representing the scientific research cycle for contextual purposes: research outputs, knowledge transfer, clinical implementation, community benefit, policy and legislation, and economic benefit. There was overlap among pathways as some indicators are applicable under multiple pathways.

A framework was constructed from the list of impact indicators and made publicly available via the Becker Library website, "Assessing the Impact of Research," to serve as a practical, do-it-yourself, web-based tool for tracking the impact of biomedical research.[13] The first edition of the website was launched in 2009 followed by a revision in 2012.[14] The website content is governed under a Creative Commons Attribution-Noncommercial-Share Alike 3.0 United States License. Users are free to copy, distribute, display, and adapt the content as noted on the website for noncommercial purposes as long as attribution is provided to Becker Library.

The framework of impact indicators is intended to help provide clues or examples to create a narrative of impact beyond publication and citation data as an aid to help with research reporting. Guidance for quantifying and documenting each impact indicator was also developed and made available on the website.

The 2012 website version (current version) contains a list of impact indicators categorized into five pathways:

- Advancement of knowledge;
- Clinical implementation;
- Community benefit;
- Legislation and policy; and
- Economic benefit.

The list of impact indicators is undergoing revision to organize the content in a relational database to enable search capabilities and facilitate sustainability of the content. Additional pathways based on the scientific research cycle are planned as are definitions and a set of recommended practices for locating evidence to establish a connection between a specific impact indicator and a research study or investigator.

Application to the Clinical and Translational Science Awards

In hindsight the project was auspicious as it dovetailed with the launch of a new NIH award program, the NIH Clinical and Translational Science Awards (CTSAs), which are administered by the National Center for Advancing Translational Sciences.[15] The consortium was created to transform clinical and translational research to provide new treatments more efficiently and quickly, one of the key objectives of the NIH Roadmap for Medical Research. Institutions with CTSAs are required to have an evaluative component to assess the progress of local, translational research activities.

This requirement provides libraries with an ideal platform to demonstrate their expertise with bibliometric-based methods for evaluation of research productivity and performance. These methods require collection and validation of publication data including reconciling author variants and knowledge of appropriate bibliometric analyses.

The OHTS project helped Becker Library acquire new skill sets that resulted into being appointed to the tracking and evaluation team at Washington University's CTSA, the Institute for Clinical and Translational Science (ICTS), in 2011. Examples of services for ICTS include annual publication and citation reports for ICTS members; reconciliation of author name variants found in databases; recommendations of bibliometric analyses to highlight productivity and performance; development of a collection for ICTS publications in the library's institutional repository, Digital Commons@Becker;[16] and identification of impact from ICTS-funded research for reporting purposes, to name a few. The overarching goal of these services is to help ICTS produce meaningful narratives of translational health outcomes resulting from CTSA-funded research.

Service Model: Publishing and Evaluation Support Program at Becker Library

The identification of research and publication practices during the OHTS project led to the development of a holistic workshop titled "Enhancing the Visibility and Impact of Your Research," which covers the following areas: establishing an author profile; publication tips; strategies to promote discoverability and dissemination of research findings; tracking research outputs and activities; and tips for creating a narrative about research. This workshop is now provided on a regular basis at Becker Library and is modified for specific audiences, including young investigators and scholars, clinicians, and administrators. Other workshops developed as a result of the OHTS project include the following:

- Who Is Citing Your Work?
- Selecting a Journal for Publication;
- Assessing the Impact of Your Research; and
- Using Publication Data to Measure Productivity and Impact.

The research and publication practices helped to strengthen the outreach efforts of the scholarly communications program at Becker Library established in fall 2007. These practices provided an ideal segue for support services in the areas of copyright and public access mandates and with recruiting collections for the library's institutional repository, Digital Commons@Becker.

The scholarly communications program evolved to the publishing and evaluation support program in spring 2014. Examples of services include publication and citation reports for authors and investigators with contextual narratives; supplementing promotion and tenure packets; recruiting reports; providing justification for funding applications or renewals; assisting with department and institutional benchmarking; and consultation services. One frequent service is review of funding applications and using publication data to help establish an investigator as being best qualified to undertake the research or to demonstrate a gap in the research being proposed. Likewise, a renewal for funding can be bolstered by publication data and citation data.

Another example of a frequent request is a coauthor network map to demonstrate collaboration patterns among a group of authors in a research department or special-

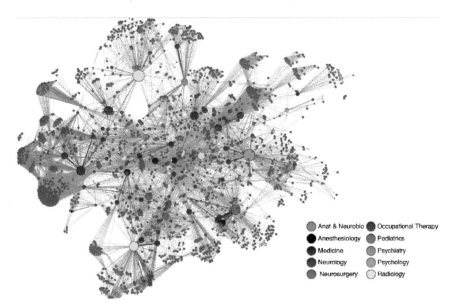

Figure 14.4.   Coauthor Network, Science of Science (Sci2) Tool. Indiana University and SciTech Strategies, http://sci2.cns.iu.edu/.

ized research center. The coauthor network map is based on publication data and allows for visualization of patterns invisible through publication data alone. Some network maps display coalescence among the authors as seen in figure 14.4; other maps show a loosely connected network or clusters that can help identify gaps in collaboration. Per Belter, visualization network services can be a valuable means of helping investigators and institutions with demonstrating the value of their research.[17] Another increasingly popular request is h-index reports for individuals and departments. The program has further expanded to include support with the new NIH Biosketch format, required as of May 25, 2015. See the "Reporting Impact Trends" section for more information on the new NIH Biosketch format.

Services are provided for authors, investigators, students, research teams, and administrators. In some instances, additional consultation is required to clarify the intended message and target audience. Sometimes a "pretty picture" is not the most appropriate means of conveying a specific message for an intended purpose. We also work to establish clear communication with our clients to manage expectations to avoid any surprises or disappointment. All reports include disclaimers as to data sources, especially if from bibliographic databases (see textbox 14.4).

Another key component of our program efforts is discretion. Drafts of funding proposals are sent to the library for review as well as information requests for recruitment or tenure purposes that contain highly sensitive information. We emphasize that requests and delivered work products remain confidential and will not be shared with others.

TEXTBOX 14.4
Disclaimers

The summary report is based on publication and citation data (including self-citations) from XYZ. Publication and citation data may be incomplete due to coverage and name variant issues.

While publication data can provide compelling narratives, no single metric is sufficient for measuring performance, quality, or impact by an author. Publication data alone does not provide a full overview of impact or influence, nor is it predictive of meaningful health outcomes. Publication data represents but one facet of research outputs and activities by an author. For a list of academic/research outputs and activities, see http://beckerguides.wustl.edu/impactofpublications.

We find that word of mouth is our most effective tool for promoting the new program, and information about the program is available on the library website (https://becker.wustl.edu/) and in resource guides (http://beckerguides.wustl.edu/).

There are a number of challenges with establishing and maintaining this type of service program. Starting a publishing and evaluation support program requires knowledge of evaluation methods, team science, and bibliometrics, as well as keeping track of trends and developments in reporting of research by funding agencies and institutions. A significant investment of time is required to learn new software and gain expertise, and keeping up with the literature and trends is an ongoing effort. Specific time periods are especially hectic, particularly around grant application and report dates. Managing expectations as well as other commitments can be challenging during these times. Additional challenges we face and identified by Hendrix include lack of standardization of promotion and tenure criteria among departments on a campus, the time-intensive nature of executing bibliometric analyses, and lack of staffing to perform detailed reports.[18] Despite these challenges, the program is successful, with two full-time staff members devoted to providing support with additional staff members pulled in to help with projects as needed.

APPLICABILITY TO OTHER LIBRARIES

Medical libraries offer substantial expertise in navigating the array of resources that exist to illustrate a narrative of research productivity, performance, and impact that can be transmuted into innovative programs aligned with institutional needs. Among the expertise and skill sets held by libraries are bibliographic database management; retrieval and analysis of data; understanding of author/affiliation ambiguity issues; knowledge of publication patterns by authors and investigators; and knowledge of the scientific research process including funding mechanisms, to name a few.[19,20,21,22] Some libraries have staff with expertise in bibliometrics. Per Bladek, bibliometrics is one of the key skill sets that libraries can use to parlay their expertise into "forming a well-informed approach to research assessment at their institution."[23] Other libraries are generating network maps using social network analysis.[24] Such efforts are subject to increased complexity but nonetheless hold promise in strengthening the role of the library among campus partners.[25] Evaluation to assess productivity and impact can occur at the individual author level; the department level; the research group level, including physical or virtual research groups; the institutional level; or for a transient population such as scholars/trainees in which longitudinal tracking is required for reporting purposes. Some strategies for getting started are noted in textbox 14.5.

TEXTBOX 14.5
Strategies for Libraries Considering Evaluation Services

- Capitalize on serendipity; sometimes the best opportunities are simply a result of happenstance.
- Consider your current campus connections: Can they help make new connections? Can they identify gaps or needs that the library can address? Can they offer solutions or a plan?
- Ask specific research groups what their criteria is for performance reviews.
- Can the library piggyback with an existing service model?
- Start small with a single service such as publication and citation reports. Post examples of publication reports that can be done for authors or research groups.
- Learn a new skill set if there is a need for a particular resource or service.
- Partner with campus groups that track university performance for benchmarking purposes or need to provide information to university ranking organizations.
- Become familiar with the literature on bibliometrics and evaluation.
- Adopt a "did you know approach" to allow for subtle introduction to resources and services.
- Become familiar with campus promotion and tenure requirements and develop resources to help individuals with their tenure/promotion packet.
- Identify campus research trends over time.
- Learn new software tools such as Sci2 (https://sci2.cns.iu.edu/user/index.php), NodeXL (http://nodexl.codeplex.com/), or Publish or Perish (http://www.harzing.com/pop.htm).

REPORTING IMPACT TRENDS

Changes in the landscape toward reporting of research are evident; academic institutions and funding agencies in the United States place a growing emphasis on acknowledging other work products besides traditional journal articles and are moving toward measures that provide tangible outcomes such as knowledge diffusion, synthesis into clinical applications, and influence on public policy. Using numbers, or "counts," based on productivity and impact (number of publications, number of citations, journal impact factor scores, etc.) is no longer sufficient to demonstrate a return on investment, nor is it meaningful for nonacademic audiences.

Funding agencies have been among organizations focusing on more meaningful metrics for reporting of research. The National Science Foundation's (NSF) "Biographical Sketch" includes a section titled "Synergistic Activities" to allow for listing of examples that demonstrate the broader impact of an individual's professional and scholarly activities.[26] NSF was also among the first to note a change in the focus from the journal article as being the sole research product to include other forms of "products" such as data sets, software, patents, and copyrights.[27] The publications section was renamed as the products section. Examples include:

- Innovations in teaching and training;
- Contributions to the science of learning;
- Development or refinement of research tools;
- Computation methodologies and algorithms for problem solving;
- Development of databases to support research and education;
- Broadening the participation of groups underrepresented in science, mathematics, engineering, and technology; and
- Service to the scientific and engineering community outside of the individual's immediate organization.

The new NIH Biosketch requires investigators to provide up to five narratives describing their contributions to science and, for each contribution, to list up to four peer-reviewed publications including nonpublication research products such as audio or video products, patents, data and research materials, databases, educational aids or curricula, instruments or equipment, models, protocols, and software.[28]

The contributions to science narratives represent a focus on accomplishments, not publications, and allow for discussion of roles played in scientific discoveries and their significance. The new NIH Biosketch is required for NIH and AHRQ applications as of May 25, 2015.

The Centers for Disease Control (CDC) has developed a framework for public health to demonstrate how CDC Science is making a difference.[29] The Science Impact Framework can be used prospectively or retrospectively and utilizes indicators to measure impact toward health outcomes, through five levels of influence: disseminating science, creating awareness, catalyzing action, effecting change, and shaping the future. The National Institute of Environmental Health Sciences (NIEHS) has implemented strong evaluation programs that emphasize reporting of qualitative-based outcomes and produced a manual, *Partnerships for Environmental Public Health: Evaluation Metrics Manual*, which emphasizes harmonized reporting of qualitative outcomes by Partnerships for Environmental Public Health (PEPH) grantees and program staff.[30]

Universities and research organizations are also striving to report on research efforts that transcend simple counts and are working to develop harmonized methods for assessment that illustrate meaningful outcomes. The Science and Technology for America's Reinvestment: Measuring the EffecT of Research on Innovation, Competitiveness and Science, or STAR METRICS project, launched in 2010, is an example of this effort.[31] STAR METRICS is an effort led by the NIH and the NSF under the auspices of Office of Science and Technology Policy (OSTP), in collaboration with research organizations and universities. The objectives for STAR METRICS are to establish uniform and auditable measures of the impact of science spending and to develop measures of impact on scientific knowledge, social outcomes, workforce outcomes, and economic growth.

Professional societies and organizations are also emphasizing the need for improving the methods of evaluating and reporting on impact from scientific research. The San Francisco Declaration on Research Assessment (DORA) resulted from a conference of the American Society for Cell Biology in 2012.[32] DORA includes a set of recommendations urging funding bodies, publishers, and institutions to avoid use of the Journal Citation Reports Impact Factor score as a means of assessing research impact or scientific quality. DORA also encourages others to think beyond the journal article as the primary metric for research output to include other outputs such as data sets and software, and to consider qualitative indicators such as influence on policy and practice. Among other metrics for evaluation research suggested by DORA are article-level metrics, the scientific content of a publication, the influence of a work on policy and practice, and the h-index.

DORA was followed by a statement from the Institute of Electrical and Electronics Engineers (IEEE).[33] The IEEE statement, "Appropriate Use of Bibliometric Indicators for the Assessment of Journals, Research Proposals, and Individuals," contains a set of recommendations for proper assessment of works in the fields of engineering, computer science, and information technology. Among the recommendations are that multiple indicators are required for evaluation purposes and that a journal-based metric should not be used as a proxy for single-article quality or to evaluate individual scientists.

These trends as well as others are relevant for medical libraries that may be considering establishing a program for evaluation services. Libraries should monitor the environment to ensure that evaluation programs are aligned with the changing needs of scholars and investigators.[20] Other trends that can be capitalized by libraries include leveraging features offered by bibliographic databases to help with evaluation; assisting with article-level metrics and their applicability for reporting of impact purposes; and applying new methods of graphically representing data.

SUMMARY

In hindsight, the retrospective analysis project and its ripple effects were serendipitous. The realization that a citation report should only be the start of any project that involves assessment of scientific productivity or performance was a pivotal point for Becker Library. The Assessing the Impact of Research website, the appointment to the ICTS tracking and evaluation team, and the new Publishing and Evaluation Support Program were not planned in advance, or even envisioned. Their creation and success were a matter of being at the right place at the right time, coupled with Becker Library's willingness to explore the development of a program to meet the needs of authors in the face of the changing landscape toward sharing and reporting of scientific research.

ACKNOWLEDGMENTS

The authors wish to acknowledge Dr. Mae Gordon's ongoing support to Becker Library. Her innate curiosity and determination were key components to the success of the retrospective analysis project. Gordon's questions continue to serve as the driving force for Becker Library efforts related to research impact.

RESOURCES

Three Zotero groups (https://www.zotero.org/) containing readings related to impact:

- Publication Assessment: https://www.zotero.org/groups/publication_assessment
- Research Impact: https://www.zotero.org/groups/research_impact
- Research Models and Frameworks: https://www.zotero.org/groups/research_modelframeworks

NOTES

1. Washington University School of Medicine in St. Louis. Ophthalmology and Visual Sciences. http://ophthalmology.wustl.edu/. Accessed February 13, 2015.
2. Sieving PC. The impact of NEI-funded multi-center trials: Bibliometric indications of dissemination, acceptance and implementation of trial findings. *Invest Ophthalmol Vis Sci.* 2007;48 E-abstract 2389. http://abstracts.iovs.org/cgi/content/abstract/48/5/2389. Accessed November 7, 2014.
3. Wells R, Whitworth JA. Assessing outcomes of health and medical research: Do we measure what counts or count what we can measure? *Aust New Zealand Health Policy.* 2007 Jun 28;4:14. doi:10.1186/1743-8462-4-14. Accessed January 21, 2015.
4. Agency for Healthcare Research and Quality (AHRQ). National Guideline Clearinghouse (NGC). http://www.guideline.gov/. Accessed February 13, 2015.
5. American Medical Association. Current Procedural Terminology (CPT). http://www.ama-assn.org/ama/pub/physician-resources/solutions-managing-your-practice/coding-billing-insurance/cpt.page. Accessed February 13, 2015.

6. Thimons JJ. Pachymetry: The new standard of care in glaucoma. *Optometric Management.* May 1, 2006. http://www.optometricmanagement.com/articleviewer.aspx?articleid=71637. Accessed February 12, 2015.

7. Murphy J. National Panel: OHTS affects when optometrists treat glaucoma. *Review of Optometry.* 2003 Jul 15;140(7).

8. Sarli CC, Dubinsky EK, Holmes KL. Beyond citation analysis: A model for assessment of research impact. *J Med Libr Assoc.* 2010 Jan;98(1):17–23. doi:10.3163/1536-5050.98.1.008. Accessed January 21, 2015.

9. Sibbald SL, MacGregor JCD, Surmacz M, Wathen CN. Into the gray: A modified approach to citation analysis to better understand research impact. *J Med Libr Assoc.* 2015;103(1):49–54. doi:10.3163/1536-5050.103.1.010. Accessed February 10, 2015.

10. Washington University School of Medicine in St. Louis. Vision Research Coordinating Center (VRCC). https://vrcc.wustl.edu/ohtsbibliography.pdf. Accessed May 6, 2015.

11. Database of Genotypes and Phenotypes (dbGaP). National Center for Biotechnology Information, U.S. National Library of Medicine. http://www.ncbi.nlm.nih.gov/gap. Accessed February 15, 2015.

12. National Library of Medicine. Authorship in MEDLINE®. National Institutes of Health, Health and Human Services. http://www.nlm.nih.gov/pubs/factsheets/authorship.html. Accessed February 13, 2015.

13. Bernard Becker Medical Library, Washington University School of Medicine in St. Louis. Assessing the impact of research. https://becker.wustl.edu/impact-assessment. Accessed February 15, 2015.

14. Sarli CC, Holmes KL. Update to beyond citation analysis: A model for assessment of research impact. *J Med Libr Assoc.* 2012 Apr;100(2):82. doi:10.3163/1536-5050.100.2.002. Accessed February 10, 2015.

15. National Institutes of Health, Health and Human Services. National Center for Advancing Translational Sciences. http://www.ncats.nih.gov/research/cts/ctsa/ctsa.html. Accessed February 13, 2015.

16. Bernard Becker Medical Library, Washington University School of Medicine in St. Louis. Digital Commons@Becker. http://digitalcommons.wustl.edu/. Accessed February 15, 2015.

17. Belter C. Visualizing networks of scientific research. *Online Magazine.* 2012;36(3):14–19.

18. Hendrix D. Tenure metrics: Bibliometric education and services for academic faculty. *Med Ref Serv Q.* 2010;29(2):183–89.

19. Drummond R, Wartho R. RIMS: The research impact measurement service at the University of New South Wales. *Aust Acad Res Libr.* 2009;40(2):76–87.

20. Drummond R. RIMS Revisited: The evolution of the research impact measurement service at UNSW library. *Aust Acad Res Libr.* 2014;45(4):309–22.

21. Bladek M. Bibliometrics services and the academic library: Meeting the emerging needs of the campus community. *College and Undergraduate Libraries.* 2014;21(3–4):330–34.

22. Corrall S, Kennan M, Afzal W. Bibliometrics and research data management services: Emerging trends in library support for research. *Library Trends.* 2013;61(3):636–74.

23. Bladek M. Bibliometrics services and the academic library: Meeting the emerging needs of the campus community. *College and Undergraduate Libraries.* 2014;21(3–4):330–34, p. 332.

24. Hunt J, Whipple E, McGowan J. Use of social network tools to validate a resources infrastructure for interinstitutional translational research: A case study. *J. Med Libr Assoc.* 2012;100(1):48–54.

25. Åström F, Hansson J. How implementation of bibliometric practice affects the role of academic libraries. *J Librariansh Inf Sci.* 2013;45(4):316–22.

26. National Science Foundation. Proposal preparation instructions; 2004. http://www.nsf.gov/pubs/gpg/nsf04_23/2.jsp. Accessed February 13, 2015.

27. National Science Foundation. Grant proposal guide summary of changes; 2013. http://www.nsf.gov/pubs/policydocs/pappguide/nsf13001/gpg_sigchanges.jsp. Accessed February 13, 2015.

28. Update: New biographical sketch format required for NIH and AHRQ grant applications submitted for due dates on or after May 25, 2015. National Institutes of Health, U.S. Department of Health and Human Services. http://grants.nih.gov/grants/guide/notice-files/NOT-OD-15-032.html. Accessed February 13, 2015.

29. Centers for Disease Control and Prevention. Advancing excellence and integrity of CDC Science. http://www.cdc.gov/od/science/impact. Accessed February 15, 2015.

30. The National Institute of Environmental Health Sciences. *Partnerships for Environmental Public Health: Evaluation Metrics Manual.* 2012. http://www.niehs.nih.gov/research/supported/assets/docs/a_c/complete_peph_evaluation_metrics_manual_508.pdf. Accessed February 15, 2015.

31. U.S. Department of Health and Human Services. STAR METRICS. https://www.starmetrics.nih.gov/. Accessed February 15, 2015.

32. The American Society for Cell Biology. San Francisco Declaration on Research Assessment. http://am.ascb.org/dora. Accessed February 15, 2015.

33. Institute of Electrical and Electronics Engineers (IEEE). Appropriate use of bibliometric indicators for the assessment of journals, research proposals, and individuals; 2013. http://www.ieee.org/publications_standards/publications/rights/ieee_bibliometric_statement_sept_2013.pdf. Accessed February 15, 2015.

15

Research Impact Assessment

Karen E. Gutzman

INTRODUCTION

The Northwestern University Clinical and Translational Sciences (NUCATS) Institute, founded in 2007, serves as a source for Clinical and Translational Science (CTS) support and funding for Northwestern University and its clinical partners. Northwestern University's Galter Library has numerous successful initiatives in support of clinical and translational science, including those detailed in chapter 2 of this book. In 2014, the library began planning a comprehensive suite of services related to research evaluation and impact assessment. The library felt that organizing research evaluation efforts into a service model and offering new, related services would greatly benefit CTS researchers and clinicians. Before I provide an example of our services, I thought it would be helpful to begin with a general overview of research evaluation. My hope is that this information is useful to librarians looking to increase their involvement in evaluation services.

Though academic libraries have traditionally been active in the field of bibliometrics for collection management and journal evaluation,[1] evidence suggests it has been combined with other techniques for research evaluation and impact assessment purposes in library services.[2] The idea of academic libraries providing services in this area has been extensively suggested[1,3,4] and successfully implemented,[5–9] but there are relatively few case studies available to document these services in the United States. Perhaps one reason for the relative lack of literature is that many libraries offer these services in specific circumstances, making only the sparsest evidence available for publication.

Some of the most confounding aspects for a librarian working in research evaluation and impact assessment include new terminologies and often confusing concepts; the deluge of messy data and paradoxically the scarcity of helpful data; idiosyncrasies of databases and data sources; the formidable challenge of analysis; and the looming possibility of unmet expectations of stakeholders regarding the scope of work or the final product. While these are practical concerns that should be considered, there is much to be gained from this area of service as well, as this type of service enables the library to better understand the needs of researchers and institutions, more fully promote and leverage expensive library resources, attract the thoughtful attention of university administrators to the capability of library staff, and so much more.

Research evaluation and impact assessment are often used interchangeably; in this chapter we will consider impact assessment as one approach for evaluating research. The following case study explains the nature of research evaluation and impact assessment and gives an example of library services in this area. The library service example at the end of the chapter is called out in the text when it pertains to the topic being discussed.

WHY EVALUATE RESEARCH?

Recent fiscal sequestration policies implemented by the U.S. government have led to an even greater need for accountability when investing taxpayer money into research. Funding agencies, institutions, policy makers, and even researchers in the United States and around the world have been pressed to explain how research has led to meaningful impact. Clinical and translational science has not been immune to this growing trend.

Guthrie and colleagues have broadly defined four key rationales for evaluating research, which are noted in figure 15.1. These rationales were developed to "understand how research can and should be evaluated in different contexts and to meet different needs."[10]

These rationales serve as aims for the evaluation process, though they may not match every situation perfectly. Below are specific examples of stakeholders and their reasons for evaluating research:

- Researchers may need to demonstrate impact of published works to promotion or tenure committees or the impact of their research studies to funding agencies when applying for future funding requests.
- Funding agencies may want to analyze why a research study failed to produce meaningful impacts in order to help future funding efforts avoid pitfalls and yield more successful results. Conversely, they may use this evidence as an advocacy tool, demonstrating to donors how increased support could provide meaningful impact to address societal health disparities.

Advocacy: to demonstrate the benefits of supporting research, enhance understanding of research and its processes among policymakers and the public; to make the case for policy and practice change.

Accountability: to show that money has been used efficiently and effectively, and hold researchers to account.

Analysis: to understand how and why research is effective and how it can be better supported, feeding into research strategy and decision-making by providing a stronger evidence base.

Allocation: to determine where best to allocate funds in the future, making the best use possible of a limited funding pot.

Figure 15.1. Key rationales for evaluation of research.

- Politicians or policy makers may need to quantify a return on investment from a newly instituted policy or funded research program.
- Academic institutions may want to analyze the workflow of successful research studies in order to better support the necessary infrastructure used by those studies. They may also want to discover how findings from their researchers are being used to promote better health outcomes.
- Patients or the public may want to understand how the research studies in which they participate inform or affect the health outcomes in their communities.

Given the broad range of stakeholders and their unique interests, it is nearly impossible to fulfill all expectations in one evaluation. Instead, the rationale for the evaluation should be realistic and should be agreed upon by all stakeholders from the onset.

WHAT DOES EVALUATION ENTAIL?

An evaluation program can be as simple or as complex as necessary, and there are many tools available to aid the process. Logic models are one of the most basic tools used in evaluation because they provide a visual description of a program agreed upon by all stakeholders. A logic model is a basic diagram of how a program

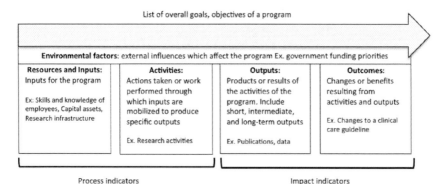

Figure 15.2.   An example of a basic logic model.

will work under specific conditions. According to Wholey, logic models have been around since the late 1960s and can be used "to evaluate a program during its design phase, after it has ended, or at any other point in its life cycle."[11]

Figure 15.2 shows an example of a traditional "cause and effect" logic model that describes how the available resources (also known as inputs) and program activities will lead to desired outputs and outcomes (both of which can be measured in the short, intermediate, or long term), given a specific environmental context.

When evaluating a program, it is useful to obtain consensus from stakeholders about the requirements of running the program (e.g., resources and inputs), how the program will accomplish its purpose (e.g., activities), the end results of the program (e.g., outputs and outcomes), and how the external environment may affect the program (e.g., environmental factors). Additionally, achieving stakeholder agreement on the overall purposes of the program, in the form of goals or objectives, is helpful.

While logic models are not always necessary for an evaluation, they do provide a flexible construct that can be used to organize a process, plan, program, and more. For example, a logic model can be used to describe an institutional department, an evaluation plan, or a researcher's career. Evaluation of research can happen at various points along the continuum of the logic model. In an evaluation to assess the impact of research, the focus shifts to the latter half of the logic model: the outputs and outcomes.

Outputs and Outcomes

The products of research are numerous and can be classified broadly as outputs or outcomes. Outputs are "the products or results of the process."[12] Research outputs are generally tangible and more easily quantified and measured than outcomes or impacts. Outputs can be classified as primary, which are the direct results of research, and secondary, which are products that "arise because of the results of research."[13]

Table 15.1. Examples of primary and secondary research outputs and research outcomes

Primary Research Outputs	Secondary Research Outputs	Research Outcomes
Journal article	Systematic review	Better-informed public
Book chapter	Clinical guideline	Changes in clinical practice
Conference paper or poster	Governmental health policy	Increased knowledge of
Data set		disease process
Software or code		More efficient testing and
Museum exhibition		diagnostics
Patient education materials		
Scientific instrumentation,		
devices, or methods		

Research outcomes are the effects, changes, or benefits on a stakeholder group resulting from the activities and outputs[13] and are generally seen over time. Examples of primary and secondary research outputs and research outcomes are found in table 15.1.

What Is Research Impact?

Impact is a topic of great interest for many universities, researchers, and other stakeholders, and libraries are the leading edge of this information because of their knowledge of literature databases, scholarly communication issues, institutional data stores, and more. There are many available definitions of research impact. Some definitions associate impact with the effects of both the outputs and outcomes. Other definitions link impact with the effects of long-term outcomes, while yet others refer only to "effects" and then parse out areas of impact.

The United Kingdom adopted the Research Excellence Framework (REF), which defines research impact as "an effect on, change or benefit to the economy, society, culture, public policy or services, health, the environment or quality of life, beyond academia."[14]

The U.S. National Institutes of Health has also taken a comprehensive stance by suggesting broad areas in which research should be impactful: our health, economy, community, and knowledge production.[15] Further links to research impact definitions can be found in figure 15.3. For evaluations that assess research impact, the definition of impact should be one that is agreed upon by stakeholders at the beginning of the evaluative process.

Formulating an Evaluation Plan

At the most basic level, designing an evaluation is a matter of asking questions. The novice may be relieved to find that the simple question, "What do you want to know?" is an acceptable place to begin an evaluation. While there are many

- **U.S. National Institutes of Health:** http://www.nih.gov/about/impact/
- **U.S. National Science Foundation:** http://www.nsf.gov/pubs/2007/ nsf07046/nsf07046.jsp
- **Primary Health Care Research & Information Service (Australia):** http://www.phcris.org.au/ publications/catalogue.php? elibid=3236&search=research +impact
- **Economic and Social Research Council (UK):** http:// www.esrc.ac.uk/funding-and- guidance/impact-toolkit/what-how- and-why/what-is-research- impact.aspx
- **Organisation for Economic Co- operation and Development:** http://www.oecd.org/ development/peer-reviews/ 2754804.pdf

---

Figure 15.3.   Definitions of research impact.

types of evaluations, a few of which are listed in figure 15.4, many evaluations can begin by formulating a question of interest and then working the question into an specific form that can be answered by one or more metrics or indicators. See table 15.2 for an example of evaluation questions to assess the impact of a team science program at a university.

```
•       Program Evaluation
•       Process Evaluation
•       Internal Evaluation
•       Risk Analysis
•       Cost-benefit analysis
•       Continuous Improvement
•       Impact Evaluation
```

Figure 15.4.   Types of evaluations.

Table 15.2.   An example of formulating evaluation questions for a team science program

General Question	Specific Questions	Indicator or Metric	Data Source
How was the collaboration between teams successful?	Was there an increase in research outputs as a result of the collaboration?	Number of publications by team members over time	Publication data from library database
	Have the team members continued to collaborate on future projects?	Positive or negative responses in survey of team members	Survey of team members

Indicators and Metrics

Once the questions are laid out, the next step is determining how to answer those questions using some sort of measurement. The terms metric, measure, and indicator are used interchangeably in evaluation literature. At times, however, their definitions differ in subtle ways. A metric or measure can be a value that is assessed against a standard benchmark or point in time. An indicator "measures a phenomenon of interest to the evaluator . . . the phenomenon can be an input, an output, an outcome, a characteristic, or an attribute";[16] indicators aren't necessarily measured against a counterpart in assessment. For purposes of brevity, I will use the term indicator to represent indicator, metric, or measure as described above.

A common way of classifying indicators is based on the areas of the logic model they measure. As noted in figure 15.2, indicators that are chosen to measure inputs and activities are typically considered process indicators as they determine the relevance and efficiency of the "process" of a program.[17] Indicators that are chosen to measure the outputs and outcomes of a program measure the program's effectiveness and are often called impact indicators.[17] Table 15.7 in the library service example provides a list of indicators (see the third column labeled "Indicators") that can be useful for libraries entering into the realm of evaluation, including counts of a researcher's peer-reviewed articles or major studies, funding sources, and number of mentees.

Considerations for Indicators

There are considerations to keep in mind when choosing indicators for an evaluation. I'll discuss two of the biggest considerations, attribution and benchmarking, below; several others are described in table 15.3.

Table 15.3.   Considerations when choosing indicators

Issue	Definition	Example
Access to data	Some data is available but not easily accessible to evaluators.	Personally identifiable information from a human resources department
Feasibility of data collection	Some data is not feasible to collect based on cost, time, or other considerations.	Data collection that continues over several years
Outside influence or guidance	Some indicators are required by outside funding agencies or groups.	Number of publications authored together by mentor and mentee
Attribution limitations	Indicators have their limits and may not be directly attributable to an outcome. Care should be taken to choose several indicators to assist in understanding the multifaceted nature of outcomes.	Attributing success of trainees based only on the positive performance feedback from a mentor
Benchmarking	Not all indicators can be assessed against a standard measurement. Sometimes data is insufficiently available or not appropriate to align with a comparison group.	Comparing the h-index of clinical researchers with those of physicists
Standardized indicators	Many indicators have proven useful over time and may be considered gold standards regardless of their perceived strengths or faults.	Using the number of publications over time to determine productivity of a researcher

While counting the total number of publications over time can tell us something about the productivity of a researcher's career, it does not provide a complete picture. This number does not tell us why one particular researcher was more productive than another, nor does it reflect a nuanced, discipline-based definition of what it means to be "successful." This is a problem of attribution: Using one indicator (e.g., high publication counts) to attribute "success" is problematic when multiple factors could be at play. An indicator generally acts as a proxy to the real story, and all indicators have their limitations. Evaluators should be aware of these limitations so they avoid "stretching the truth" of the data by assigning attribution to one factor when many factors may have contributed.

Additionally, indicators bring the problem of benchmarking: What standard is an indicator being measured or assessed against, if any at all? (As mentioned before, metrics generally have a benchmark against which they are compared.) For example, vendors of citation databases often provide research management platforms that formulate benchmarks based on curated groupings of faculty members. These platforms can be very helpful but are often expensive. While there may be a few libraries with trained evaluation staff to provide sophisticated analysis of and comparison to benchmarks for these outputs and outcomes, many library service models do not extend this far. Additionally, there are options for formulating benchmarks given access to literature databases, but it is often time consuming and requires advanced understanding of the opportunities and challenges presented by the data.

Data Collection, Sources, and Use

Many library resources, both commercial and those freely accessible, provide publication data that can contribute to or fulfill the indicators of an evaluation. Table 15.4 provides a small sample of data sources and examples of data that can be collected. Some commercial data sources provide data analysis through upgraded services to existing platforms, though the corresponding increase in cost may not be feasible for all libraries. Libraries with limited budgets can take advantage of data from commercialized sources that have been analyzed and made freely available. One such example is Thomson Reuters's Highly Cited Researchers (highlycited.com), which analyzes and presents the top 1 percent most highly cited researchers in a field using data from the Essential Science Indicators product.

Additionally, libraries should not underestimate the use of freely available data. The scholarly database from the University of Indiana provides an online interface to six databases, including National Institutes of Health and National Science Foundation funding, MEDLINE, and U.S. Patent and Trademark Office patents. While the database does require registration for use, it provides a free and useful way to search across databases.

Finally, with some ingenuity, libraries can transform the plethora of accessible bibliographic data into helpful metrics. For example, Thomson Reuters's Web of Science

Table 15.4. Examples of data sources

Data Source	Availability	Sample of Data Available
Elsevier's Scopus	Commercial	List of country affiliations of citing authors for a researcher's articles
		Top keywords used for a researcher's articles
Thomson Reuters's Web of Science	Commercial	List of second-generation citing papers
		List of papers in a predefined research category
Thomson Reuters's Essential Science Indicators	Commercial	List of hot or highly cited papers by researcher
		Emerging research fronts
Google Scholar	Free	H-index that may include more than peer-reviewed literature
		Number of research outputs over time
Scholarly Database	Free, requires registration	Researchers funded by NIH grants
		U.S. patents filed by researchers
NIH RePORTER	Free	List of articles that have cited a relevant grant
Highly Cited Researchers (by Thomson Reuters)	Free	List of researchers ranking in the top 1 percent most cited for their subject field and year of publication

(WOS) has predefined research categories that are generally assigned at the journal level. If the evaluation question is designed to demonstrate a research group's overall impact in an area of science, search WOS based on the relevant research category, limit to the intended years, and search within the top hundred (or some other predefined number) cited articles for works authored by the research group of interest. This type of data may not be of interest to all evaluators but serves as an example of how to be creative with available resources.

The library may also see fit to employ additional means of data collection, including interviews, surveys, in-depth case studies, alternative metrics (e.g., altmetrics) and more to supplement data they've already collected. Below are a few helpful publications regarding tools for research evaluation:

• Guthrie and colleagues provide a great overview of case studies, data mining, and economic analysis and more in the appendices of their report on measuring research.[10]
• Neylon and colleagues discuss altmetrics in detail, using the context of institutions in sub-Saharan Africa.[18]
• Carpenter and colleagues examine citation analysis, give lists of descriptors of publication data, and discuss indices for measuring productivity.[19]

There are so many helpful resources and tools available that keeping up with trends in this area can be challenging. As suggested later in this chapter, there are many groups dedicated to furthering research evaluation and impact assessment; participating in these groups provides opportunities to learn about resources and tools from a wide-reaching community of evaluators.

Table 15.5. Examples of evaluation frameworks

Research Excellence Framework (REF), UK	http://www.ref.ac.uk/
Excellence in Research for Australia (ERA), AU	http://www.arc.gov.au/era
Star Metrics, US	https://www.starmetrics.nih.gov/
Balanced Scorecard	https://balancedscorecard.org/
Becker Model for Assessment of Research Impact	https://becker.wustl.edu/impact-assessment
Canadian Academy of Health Sciences (CAHS) Impact Framework	http://www.cahs-acss.ca/making-an-impact-a-preferred-framework-and-indicators-to-measure-returns-on-investment-in-health-research-8
Metrics Champion Consortium (MCC)	http://metricschampion.org/

Evaluation Frameworks

Logic models are not the only method for approaching evaluation in a systematic fashion. Many successful frameworks can inform or enhance an evaluation plan. Two relevant frameworks are the Becker Model for Assessment of Research Impact, which is a list of indicators of impact, and the Canadian Academy of Health Sciences (CAHS) Impact Framework, which consists of a logic model and an extensive list of indicators. Several other frameworks are listed in table 15.5. Guthrie and colleagues published a helpful comparison of several of these frameworks.[10]

The Becker Model for Assessment of Research Impact was developed in 2009 at Washington University in St. Louis's Becker Medical Library by Cathy Sarli, Kristi Holmes, and Ellen Dubinsky.[9] The model designates five areas of research impact: advancement of knowledge, clinical implementation, community benefit, legislation and policy, and economic benefit. Each area has a host of indicators, with the entire model consisting of more than three hundred indicators. It may be helpful to review these indicators when formulating evaluation questions and assigning indicators. More information on the Becker Model is available in chapter 14 of this book.

The CAHS Impact Framework, funded by twenty-three organizations and published in 2009, is a standard for evaluating the impacts of health research in Canada. This framework consists of a logic model that serves as a "road map" for tracking health research impacts in five main categories: "advancing knowledge, building capacity, informing decision-making, health impacts, and broad socio-economic impacts."[13] Along with the logic model is a bank of indicators that are classified according to the level of analysis: the individual, group/program/grant, institution, and national.

Both the Becker Model and the CAHS framework are freely accessible online and serve as launching points for research evaluation and impact assessment that can be utilized in many situations.

Communicating with Stakeholders

Often the most important aspect of providing services in research evaluation and impact assessment is communicating the results to stakeholders. One particularly

Table 15.6.   Examples of visualization tools

Visualization Tools	Availability	Examples of Visualizations
Sci2 Tool	Free	Time-series plots, choropleth maps, proportionate symbol maps, burst analysis, radial tree graphs, social networks
Tableau	Commercial	Bubble charts, choropleth maps, bar and line charts
Microsoft Excel	Commercial	Trend lines, bar charts, infographics
Adobe Illustrator	Commercial	Infographics
Inkscape	Free	Infographics
Wordle	Free	Word clouds
Taxgedo	Free	Word clouds
Google Charts	Free	Line and bar charts, infographics
Diagrammer	Free	Work-flow diagrams
Pajek	Free	Social networks
Cytoscape	Free	Social networks

effective way of communicating evaluation data is to provide helpful visualizations of the information. Edward Tufte, an expert in information visualization, explains that the visualizations should convey the greatest number of ideas in the shortest time possible using the least amount of ink and the smallest space necessary. Additionally, Tufte stresses that visualizations should tell the truth of the data and not distort what the data is saying.[20]

It is important to have a cadre of visualization tools to choose from when making effective visualizations. Some available tools are listed in table 15.6 along with a few examples of the visualizations they can produce. Additionally, the library service example focuses on data visualization for impact reporting.

CTSA Evaluation Landscape

The original committee structure for the National Center for Advancing Translational Sciences (NCATS) included several key function committees (KFCs), one of which was the Evaluation KFC. In late 2014, NCATS unveiled a plan for a new structure of five domain task forces, each headed by a five-person lead team.[21] The work of evaluation falls into the Methods and Processes Domain Taskforce, which holds bimonthly calls and is allowed to have up to five working groups at any given time.

Other national groups have devoted themselves to furthering evaluation in the clinical and translational environment. The American Evaluation Association has a newly formed Translational Research Evaluation Topical Interest Group. Additionally, the Association for Clinical and Translational Science has the Translational Research Evaluation Special Interest Group. Both groups hold regular calls for their members, and the groups work collaboratively on strategies to evaluate translational research, including the development of common metrics and measures. In the library realm, the Medical Library Association (MLA) has the Translational Sciences Collaboration Special Interest Group that meets during the MLA annual conference.

Several publications of note have advanced research evaluation for clinical and translational science. This information-rich environment includes these publications:

- Dembe and colleagues have been working on a "standardized tool for identifying and measuring impacts across research sites" within the Clinical and Translational Science Awards (CTSAs). The group has identified seventy-two impact indicators and has begun field testing to determine the availability of data for each indicator.[22]
- Trochim and colleagues published a framework for evaluating the CTSA program that was the cumulative work of the Evaluation KFC.[23]
- Rubio also published the work of the Evaluation KFC, including the identification of fifteen common metrics in six categories that each CTSA institution should be able to collect in common with others.[24]
- Pincus and colleagues published a top ten list of lessons learned in CTSA evaluation.[25]
- Trochim and colleagues introduced a process marker model for evaluation that views translational research as a continuous process and distinguishes "observable points in the process that can be operationally defined and measured."[26]

LIBRARY SERVICE EXAMPLE: INFORMATION VISUALIZATION

Galter Library is uniquely situated under the organizational structure of Northwestern University's Clinical and Translational Science (NUCATS) Institute. While the library's funding is not contingent on NUCATS, the library derives many benefits from this relationship. As a partner to the success of NUCATS, the library is seen as a teammate, collaborator, and innovator in projects connected to NUCATS members. Additionally, our involvement in NUCATS provides avenues of communication to advocate for and impart information about the library's services, capabilities, and interests so that more NUCATS members can benefit.

Galter Library provides research evaluation and impact assessment services to NUCATS members and the greater medical school community. These services manifest in different ways, depending on the context, the level of support needed, and the capabilities of the staff. These services are meant to be flexible in nature and continuously undergo improvement based on successes and lessons learned. For group-based research-impact projects, we supply bibliographic metadata, suggest appropriate indicators, and summarize data into a report format.

Additionally, Galter Library is the home of NUCATS's Evaluation and Continuous Improvement (ECI) Program, which provides evaluation services for NUCATS as an organization. The ECI Program also licenses tools and resources for use by NUCATS and the university to better facilitate evaluation. Finally, much of the research evaluation and impact assessment work that does not center on NUCATS as a larger institution but instead focuses on individual NUCATS members, departments, and research groups is completed under the auspices of the library's Metrics and Impact Core (MIC). These services were arranged as a "core" because this language reflects how research services are typically packaged and delivered within our campus environment. Below is one example of a service as part of the Metrics and Impact Core.

Introduction

In September 2014, the Northwestern University Feinberg School of Medicine Department of Preventive Medicine requested the assistance of the library in creating a visual display of the career impact of Dr. Jeremiah Stamler for the recognition of his ninety-fifth birthday and his many years of service to the field of cardiovascular disease epidemiology. Many of the faculty members in the Department of Preventive Medicine are members of the Northwestern University Clinical and Translational Science Institute, and Galter Library's unique location within NUCATS allows for close proximity and mutual understanding of work.

Expectations

The celebration was to occur in early November 2014, and the planning committee wanted to review the finished products beforehand. We had a two-month time frame to see the project to its completion. We brainstormed some ideas and put together a packet of sample visualizations for the committee's review. We decided to base our visualizations around three areas: scholarly work, career achievement, and mentorship. We were careful to include only those visualizations that we thought were possible given the data available, the time frame, and our knowledge of visualization tools.

The committee was in favor of the visualizations we proposed and had some additional requests. They wanted us to focus some of our efforts on a few selected studies that Stamler was involved with, as well as his work in cardiovascular disease risk factors. They requested several deliverables including a PowerPoint presentation of the visualizations with detailed descriptions of the visualizations in the notes section and two large posters of visualizations for display during the event.

Methodology

After the initial meetings with the committee, we decided that the best division of effort was for me to create the visualizations and use my teammates for feedback and critical review of the outputs. I developed a rough outline of work (table 15.7) and began collecting data. I familiarized myself with Stamler's curriculum vitae (CV), watched an online interview with him, read through a few of his articles, and searched online for more information about his contemporaries and his field of study. I reserved one to two hours a day for one week for this preliminary work, knowing that the bulk of my time would be needed toward the end of the project in creating and cleaning up the visualizations and creating the PowerPoint presentation and posters.

Table 15.7. Evaluation questions for Dr. Jeremiah Stamler's career impact

General Question	Specific Questions	Indicators (Qualitative and Quantitative)	Data Sources	Visualization	Visualization Tools
What are some of the impacts of Stamler's career?	What have been the results of his scholarly work?	# of major research studies # of peer-reviewed articles from research studies Coauthorship network List of titles of journal articles List of titles of journals List of global affiliations of authors citing his articles	CV Scopus NIH RePORTER LexisNexis	Infographic of years of service, committees, publications citations, etc. Bubble chart of publication titles Choropleth map of country affiliations of citing authors Wordle of article titles Coauthor network Photos of early research, etc. Description of House Un-American Activities investigation, photo of title page of report	Adobe Illustrator Sci2 Tool Tableau Excel
	What major events have happened in his career?	# of years of service with NU # of publications, citations, awards, monographs, etc. Well-known quotations List of funding sources	CV YouTube (interview) LexisNexis	Timeline of career Temporal bar graph showing topical trends in publications	Adobe Illustrator Excel
	What are the results of his mentorship?	# of mentees Geographical location of mentees List of global affiliations of citing authors of the mentee's articles # of participants in ten-day seminar	CV Scopus University of Minnesota archive	Geographical map depicting location of trainees Choropleth map of country affiliations of citing authors to trainee articles Photo of the first ten-day seminar series	Adobe Illustrator Sci2 Tool Tableau Excel

I collected a list of Stamler's publications using Elsevier's Scopus and exported the metadata using the "export refine" feature in Scopus. I researched his brief encounter with the House Un-American Activities Committee using LexisNexis and investigated his work with the ten-day seminar series. I found an online archive from the University of Minnesota on the "History of Cardiovascular Disease Epidemiology," and I contacted one of the curators for photos of interest, especially those of the ten-day seminar series. For Stamler's major research studies, I searched for articles he authored and created timelines and summaries of these studies based on the information from the articles. I also downloaded and reviewed the Becker Model for Assessment of Research Impact to broaden my awareness of where impactful information might be found. Because this process was not a formal evaluation of Stamler's work, there would be no formal benchmarking required. Instead we focused on gathering information that would emphasize his collaborations and collegiality. During this information-gathering process, I made sure to document my work extensively so that I could verify or re-create any of my findings if needed. I tracked my progress and stored information in a Microsoft Word document, which included helpful links, dates that I visited websites, and snippets of information.

Results: Data Visualization

Once the data had been collected, I was ready to begin working on the visualizations. I reserved approximately two weeks to create the visualizations, mostly because I was unfamiliar with Adobe Illustrator and knew I would be learning how to use the program as I went along.

During this process, I kept in mind that the visualizations would need to be (a) legible in a PowerPoint presentation and (b) striking enough to garner attention on a poster. I extensively documented the workflows used to create each visualization so that they could be easily reproduced if needed. Additionally, I made sure each visualization was accompanied by a narrative section that told a short story about the visualization, emphasizing Stamler's incredible success based on his strong work ethic, his collaborations with wonderful colleagues, and his inspiring trainees. I also included a details section to allow for verification and replication of the visualization.

After the visualizations were created, we sent samples to the committee for review. Once we incorporated their comments and feedback, I took a few more days to pull the visualizations into a PowerPoint presentation and create the two posters for the event. These were once again sent to the committee for feedback and revised as necessary. We sent the finalized PowerPoint to the master of ceremonies for the event and had the two posters printed.

Following is a subset of visualizations created for the event, grouped according to Stamler's scholarly work, career achievements, and mentorship. Also included are the narrative and details sections for each visualization. Figures 15.5, 15.6, and 15.7 show scholarly work; figures 15.8 and 15.9 show career achievements; and figure 15.10 shows mentorship.

Narrative	
From his beginnings at Northwestern University as an Assistant Professor in the Department of Medicine in 1958, Dr. Stamler has given over 50 years of service, served on countless committees, and been gifted with numerous honors and awards. In addition he has guided and taught 34 trainees, and mentored countless others.	
Details	
Visualization Type:	Infographic
Topic(s):	Years of service, committees, honors and awards, trainees
Data Source(s):	Dr. Stamler's CV
Visualization Tool(s):	Adobe Illustrator
Data Span:	1944-2014
Notes:	Icons were obtained from Freepik

Figure 15.5. Infographic depicting Stamler's scholarly work.

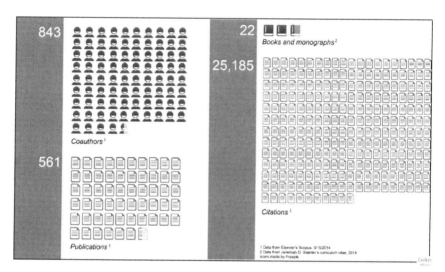

Narrative	
Dr. Stamler's contributions to the scholarly literature are numerous, with 561 publications in Elsevier's Scopus database which is the largest abstract and citation database of peer-reviewed literature. The actual total of publications of all types, numbers somewhere over 1000. Within these 561 peer-reviewed publications, Dr. Stamler has collaborated with over 843 co-authors, and has generated over 25,185 citations.	
Details	
Visualization Type:	Infographic
Topic(s):	Co-authorship, publications, citations, books and monographs
Data Source(s):	Dr. Stamler's CV and Elsevier's Scopus
Visualization Tool(s):	Adobe Illustrator
Data Span:	1944-2014
Notes:	Icons were obtained from Freepik

Figure 15.6. Infographic depicting Stamler's scholarly work.

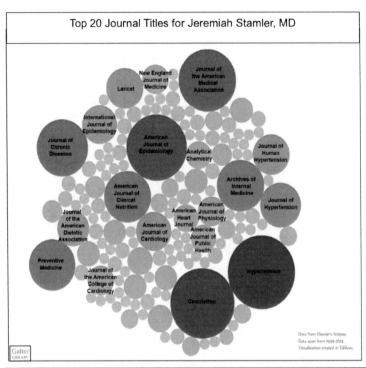

Top 20 Journal Titles for Jeremiah Stamler, MD

Narrative	
Dr. Stamler has published in many highly ranked journals, including those known for their broad coverage such as the Journal of the American Medical Association, and the Lancet, and in journals known for their cross disciplinary approach, such as Preventive Medicine, and the Journal of Chronic Diseases. Additionally, he has published in more specialized journals, such as the Journal of Human Hypertension, Hypertension and so on. Based on data from Elsevier's Scopus, he has 43 publications in Hypertension, 39 publications in Circulation, and 35 publications in the American Journal of Epidemiology. These journal titles represent a diverse audience of readers, including those interested in dietetics and nutrition, treatment of cardiovascular diseases, and preventive medicine.	

Details	
Visualization Type:	Bubble chart
Topic(s):	Analysis of journal titles published in by Dr. Stamler
Data Source(s):	Elsevier's Scopus
Visualization Tool(s):	Tableau (for the bubble chart), Adobe Illustrator (for the formatting)
Data Span:	1949-2014
Notes:	All bubbles, even those without internal text, represent journal titles

Figure 15.7.   Bubble chart depicting Stamler's scholarly work.

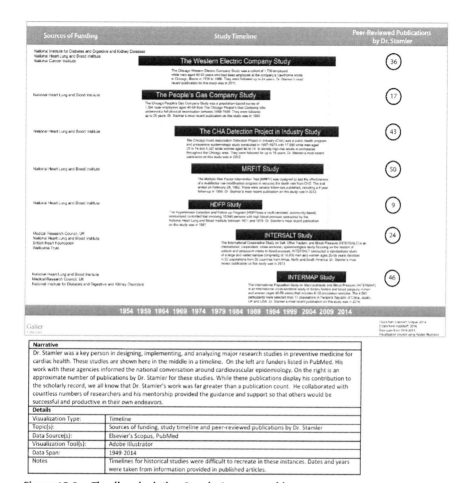

Narrative	
Dr. Stamler was a key person in designing, implementing, and analyzing major research studies in preventive medicine for cardiac health. These studies are shown here in the middle in a timeline. On the left are funders listed in PubMed. His work with these agencies informed the national conversation around cardiovascular epidemiology. On the right is an approximate number of publications by Dr. Stamler for these studies. While these publications display his contribution to the scholarly record, we all know that Dr. Stamler's work was far greater than a publication count. He collaborated with countless numbers of researchers and his mentorship provided the guidance and support so that others would be successful and productive in their own endeavors.	
Details	
Visualization Type:	Timeline
Topic(s):	Sources of funding, study timeline and peer-reviewed publications by Dr. Stamler
Data Source(s):	Elsevier's Scopus, PubMed
Visualization Tool(s):	Adobe Illustrator
Data Span:	1949-2014
Notes	Timelines for historical studies were difficult to recreate in these instances. Dates and years were taken from information provided in published articles.

Figure 15.8. Timeline depicting Stamler's career achievements.

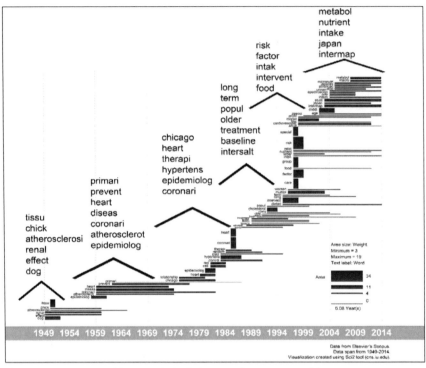

Figure 15.9.   Temporal bar graph depicting Stamler's career achievements.

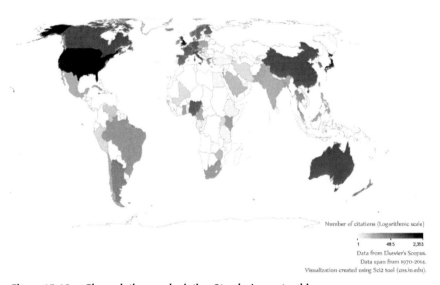

Figure 15.10.   Choropleth map depicting Stamler's mentorship.

SUCCESS, CHALLENGES, AND FUTURE WORK

The committee was pleased with the PowerPoint presentation and the two posters. The master of ceremonies chose which slides to use in the presentation and used the description and details provided with the visualizations to craft narratives that fit the overall essence of the event. We attended the event to set up the posters and to join in the evening of celebration for Stamler and his amazing work. During the event the library's work on the visualizations was recognized; this garnered attention and appreciation from the audience to the library's services in this area. We have since received several requests for information visualization work to be used in progress reports to funding agencies, alumni appreciation events, promotion and tenure packets, and so on.

The biggest challenge with this project was the necessary organization and vigilance required to document the workflows used when creating the visualizations, as well as the versions of files and sources of information, so that the visualizations could be verified or re-created if needed. A few months after the event, one of the attendees asked for a copy of the PowerPoint presentation and for information on how I created a coauthor network visualization. This request was easy to fulfill because I had been proactive about the organization of the project.

In order to maximize the benefits of this project, we decided to use the visualizations as part of a poster for a conference on visualizing data. Additionally, we have added these visualizations to a portfolio of options for any future work in this area. Moving forward, we hope to continually expand upon our skills and the visualizations we are able to create.

CONCLUSION

Research evaluation and impact assessment are crucial to the success of clinical and translational science, and the library can provide meaningful contributions in this area. By understanding the evaluation process, the motivations of stakeholders, and the types of indicators and data available, each library or librarian can find his or her own best fit in this realm. There are many types of services that can be offered based on the types of staff expertise, resources, and tools utilized by the library.

RESOURCES FOR FURTHER STUDY

Anyone interested in gaining further training or finding groups that are working in the area of research evaluation and impact assessment may find the following resources useful.

Trainings

- The American Evaluation Association (AEA) hosts a three-day Summer Evaluation Institute designed for any career stage on topics ranging from qualitative and quantitative analyses, project management, logic modeling, reporting, and more. (http://www.eval.org/p/cm/ld/fid=99)
- The International School on Research Impact Assessment is a week-long training course on measuring and assessing research impact with a focus on biomedical and health sciences. (http://www.theinternationalschoolonria.com/)
- The European Summer School for Scientometrics is a week-long training event on using scientometrics to measure and analyze trends in science and technology. (http://www.scientometrics-school.eu/index.html)
- The Cyberinfrastructure for Network Science Center hosts an Information Visualization Massive Open Online Course (MOOC) to learn more about data patterns and trends and information visualization using the Sci2 Tool. (http://cns.iu.edu/ivmooc.html)

Associations/Societies

- The International Society for Scientometrics and Infometrics (ISSI) provides communication and information exchange on the topics of scientometrics and infometrics. (http://issi-society.org/news.html)
- The Association for Computing Machinery (ACM) Special Interest Group on Performance Evaluation (SIGMETRICS) promotes performance analysis techniques, tools, and methods. (http://www.sigmetrics.org/index.shtml)
- The American Society for Information Science and Technology (ASIS&T) hosts a Metrics Special Interest Group (MET) for measurement of information production and use, including bibliometrics, scientometrics, infometrics, and visualizations. (http://www.asis.org/SIG/met.html)
- The AEA's Topical Interest Group on Translational Research Evaluation provides a community for evaluators interested in the evaluation of research. (http://comm.eval.org/translationalresearchevaluation/home)
- The Association for Clinical and Translational Science (ACTS) hosts a special interest group on translational research evaluation that focuses on evaluation techniques and methods for clinical and translational science. (http://www.actscience.org/?page=ACTSSIGS)
- The Medical Library Association's Translational Sciences Collaboration Special Interest Group provides a venue for members to share their experiences, find collaborators, and keep track of legislative or funding trends related to translational science. (http://tsc.mlanet.org/)

NOTES

1. Petersohn S. Bibliometric services in research evaluation: A new task area strengthening the jurisdiction of academic librarians. 2014. http://docs.lib.purdue.edu/iatul/2014/perfor mance/1. Accessed December 22, 2014.

2. Brown S, Key Perspectives Ltd. *A Comparative Review of Research Assessment Regimes in Five Countries and the Role of Libraries in the Research Assessment Process: A Pilot Study Commissioned by OCLC Research.* Dublin, OH: OCLC Research; 2009. http://www.oclc.org/research/ publications/library/2009/2009-09.pdf. Accessed January 22, 2015.

3. Herther NK. Research evaluation and citation analysis: Key issues and implications. *Electron Libr.* 2009;27(3):361–75. doi:10.1108/02640470910966835.

4. Åström F, Hansson J. How implementation of bibliometric practice affects the role of academic libraries. *J Librariansh Inf Sci.* 2013;45(3):316–22. doi:10.1177/0961000612456867.

5. Ball R, Tunger D. Bibliometric analysis: A new business area for information professionals in libraries? *Scientometrics.* 2013;66(3):561–77. doi:10.1007/s11192-006-0041-0.

6. Drummond R, Wartho R. RIMS: The research impact measurement service at the University of New South Wales. *Aust Acad Res Libr.* 2009;40(2):76–87.

7. Drummond R. RIMS Revisited: The evolution of the research impact measurement service at UNSW library. *Aust Acad Res Libr.* 2014;45(4):309–22. doi:10.1080/00048623.2 014.945065.

8. Hendrix D. Tenure metrics: Bibliometric education and services for academic faculty. *Med Ref Serv Q.* 2010;29(2):183–89. doi:10.1080/02763861003723416.

9. Sarli CC, Dubinsky EK, Holmes KL. Beyond citation analysis: A model for assessment of research impact. *J Med Libr Assoc.* 2010 Jan;98(1):17–23. doi:10.3163/1536-5050.98.1.008.

10. Guthrie S, Wamae W, Diepeveen S, Wooding S, Grant J. Measuring research. 2013. http://www.rand.org/pubs/monographs/MG1217.html. Accessed January 22, 2015.

11. Wholey JS. *Handbook of Practical Program Evaluation.* San Francisco: Jossey-Bass; 2010.

12. WHO. Glossary of terms used. http://www.who.int/hia/about/glos/en. Accessed January 22, 2015.

13. Panel on Return on Investment in Health Research. *Making an Impact: A Preferred Framework and Indicators to Measure Returns on Investment in Health Research.* Ottawa, Canada: Canadian Academy of Health Sciences; 2009. http://www.cahs-acss.ca/wp-content/ uploads/2011/09/ROI_FullReport.pdf. Accessed January 22, 2015.

14. *Assessment Framework and Guidance on Submissions* (updated to include addendum published in January 2012). Bristol, UK: Research Excellence Framework; 2011. http://www .ref.ac.uk/media/ref/content/pub/assessmentframeworkandguidanceonsubmissions/GOS%20 including%20addendum.pdf. Accessed January 22, 2015.

15. National Institutes of Health (NIH). Impact: About NIH. http://www.nih.gov/about/ impact. Accessed January 22, 2015.

16. Gertler PJ, Martinez S, Premand P, Rawlings LB, Vermeersch CMJ. *Impact Evaluation in Practice.* Interactive textbook at http://www.worldbank.org.pdf. Washington, DC: World Bank; 2010. http://elibrary.worldbank.org/doi/book/10.1596/978-0-8213-8541-8. Accessed January 22, 2015.

17. Graham Kenny's definition of indicators of success.

18. Neylon C, Willmers M, King T. Rethinking impact: Applying altmetrics to southern African research. 2014. https://open.uct.ac.za/handle/11427/2285. Accessed January 23, 2015.

19. Carpenter CR, Cone DC, Sarli CC. Using publication metrics to highlight academic productivity and research impact. *Acad Emerg Med.* 2014;21(10):1160–72. doi:10.1111/acem.12482.

20. Tufte ER. *The Visual Display of Quantitative Information.* Cheshire, CT: Graphics Press; 1983.

21. Domain Task Forces. https://www.ctsacentral.org/articles/domain-task-forces. Accessed January 22, 2015.

22. Dembe AE, Lynch MS, Gugiu PC, Jackson RD. The translational research impact scale development, construct validity, and reliability testing. *Eval Health Prof.* 2014;37(1):50–70. doi:10.1177/0163278713506112.

23. Trochim WM, Rubio DM, Thomas VG. Evaluation guidelines for the Clinical and Translational Science Awards (CTSAs). *Clin Transl Sci.* 2013;6(4):303–9. doi:10.1111/cts.12036.

24. Rubio DM. Common metrics to assess the efficiency of clinical research. *Eval Health Prof.* 2013;36(4):432–46. doi:10.1177/0163278713499586.

25. Pincus HA, Abedin Z, Blank AE, Mazmanian PE. Evaluation and the NIH Clinical and Translational Science Awards: A "top ten" list. *Eval Health Prof.* 2013;36(4):411–31. doi:10.1177/0163278713507061.

26. Trochim W, Kane C, Graham M, Pincus HA. Evaluating translational research: A process marker model. *Clin Transl Sci.* 2011;4(3):153–62. doi:10.1111/j.1752-8062.2011.00291.x.

16

Web Design, Evaluation, and Bibliometrics—Oh, My!

From Local CTSA Work to National Involvement

Elizabeth C. Whipple

INTRODUCTION

The Indiana CTSI (Clinical and Translational Sciences Institute) was established in 2008 and includes the state's major research universities: Indiana University (IU), Purdue University, and the University of Notre Dame. The Indiana University School of Medicine (IUSM) in Indianapolis is the home institute for the Indiana CTSI. In 2008, the director of the Ruth Lilly Medical Library (RLML) of the IUSM was named the director of the CTSI Evaluation and Tracking Program. She ensured that participation from RLML librarians was written into the grant and funded from the beginning of the project. These connections for the RLML at a high level of the CTSI organizational structure helped to ensure that medical librarians were at the table from the very beginning, with funded effort and influential collaborators already in place.

RLML librarians have been involved in several CTSI programs, including bio-medical informatics, tracking and evaluation, and the Community Health Engagement Program (CHEP). The majority of librarian efforts, including my own work, have been focused on program evaluation and development of CTSI resources. In this case study, I describe my work in two primary areas: the design and redesign of the institute's web portal and my involvement in our CTSI's Evaluation and Tracking Program, which led to my participation in a national committee and work group.

CTSI HUB

The Indiana CTSI Hub is an "online portal providing resources for research, education and collaboration in many areas of science."[1] These resources are available not only to biomedical researchers at the three partner CTSI universities but to all researchers and local and national community health organizations. Hub resources include shared contributions from the science community, commercial software products, and in-house databases. Sample resources include REDCap, a platform for data management and surveying; i2b2 (Informatics for Integrating Biology and the Bedside), a scalable informatics framework; tissue banks (the Indiana BioBank and the Susan G. Komen Tissue Bank at the IU Simon Cancer Center); GOBIOM Biomarker Database; and the Open Journal Systems software, for grant application submission. The array of tools and resources available through the hub is designed to address the needs of researchers, clinical program managers, and community organizations and members of the public who are interested and involved with clinical and translational research. The hub was developed to be much more than a website and is designed to promote and extend clinical and translational research by providing a collaborative platform for researchers, academics, commercial entities, and community groups.

The CTSI Hub is housed in and maintained by the University Information Technology Services (UITS) at IU and built on HUBzero, software developed at Purdue University. Many stakeholders within IU, Purdue, and Notre Dame were involved with the CTSI Hub group from its conception. Meeting participants included representatives from university Research Service Cores and Project Development Teams, as well as hub programmers and other CTSI program representatives from entities including CHEP and the Bioethics and Subject Advocacy Program (BSAP). Because of our skills in accessing and organizing information, the library director recommended that RLML librarians also have a seat at hub meetings. The hub group initially met to talk about issues including the usability and structure of the site, the different groups of potential users of the site, and the kinds of resources and tools that should be available through the hub.

Library representation varied but generally consisted of two others and myself. Initially we were a little unsure as to what role we could play in this group but viewed this as an opportunity to participate in discussions, hear people's concerns, and learn how others viewed the hub's primary purposes and content. It didn't take long before our expertise proved useful to the group. For example, there was extensive discussion on the hub's search box and the actual content it would search. Would it simply search across the content on the hub, or could it also search within specific parts of the hub? Some stakeholders also wanted federated search capabilities, enabling the search to retrieve results from resources such as PubMed and other government websites. We identified this as a chance to share our expertise on issues of accessibility and usability. In the case of the search box, we argued that a federated search would (1) provide unexpected or irrelevant results and (2) provide too many results. In other words, rather than enhancing discoverability, a federated search could overwhelm users and could prevent them from easily locating what they needed.

We were also able to leverage our skills when the hub explored the possibility of incorporating researcher collaboration tools. We helped to test a homegrown research collaboration tool and provided feedback for improving and tweaking the tool. This tool included setting up a personal profile, finding people to add to your network, messaging with each other, and sharing documents and other data within your team/groups. We tested these various features and gave feedback on what we liked, what worked/what didn't work, and what other features would be good to have. While this tool did not end up becoming part of the hub platform (and the creator moved to a different institution), many of the features that were part of it are standard in research collaboration tools today.

During our time on the hub committee, we developed good working relationships with other members of the committee, who began to recognize the value of our role and expertise in helping to develop and structure the hub. One major effort during this time was to identify an ontology tool for the hub. Several committee members, including all of the librarians, were interested in learning how to better structure information on the hub. We contacted the National Center for Biomedical Ontology (NCBO) to see if using their ontology tool, BioPortal, would be a useful addition to the hub and its search feature. While we ultimately decided not to incorporate the NCBO tool, it was a good exercise and a chance to demonstrate our expertise in how information can be organized, such as explaining how medical subject headings (MeSH) work and how MeSH trees are organized and accessed.

As the hub became more established, stakeholders found the hub sufficient for their needs and no longer felt the need to provide input by participating in the work of the committee. At this point, however, those of us still on the committee realized that there was a need for a site redesign because different groups of people were using the hub and for different purposes. Additionally, the CTSI administration wanted the hub to add some different functionality to enhance the process of different groups using the hub to find what they needed. A hub redesign subcommittee was designed to address these needs.

Our redesign committee consisted of a biostatistician from the Design and Biostatics Program (DBP), two medical librarians involved in the Tracking and Evaluation Program and CHEP, an academic literature specialist from the BSAP, a program manager for CHEP, and a computational astrophysicist involved with information technology/hub infrastructure from the Biomedical Informatics Program.

The subcommittee had two main goals. Our primary goal was to test the usability of the hub front page, specifically its navigation structure; our secondary goal was to gauge the effectiveness of the front-page content and its general look and feel. For these usability tests to provide meaningful and useful feedback, we had to (1) know the types of users who would likely use the hub, and (2) identify individuals who could represent those types of users and who would be willing to participate in this activity. Since we had already been working on the hub for a couple of years, we all had various contacts that we were able to enlist. We ended up with eleven volunteers representing six potential user groups (IUSM faculty, community organization representatives, graduate students, information-technology staff, a non-IUSM physician, and a couple of adolescents).

As librarians, we are familiar with using the card-sort procedure to determine users' experience with the website. In a card-sort activity, you identify the concepts that currently exist within a website, write them down on cards (or sticky notes), and then ask users to arrange them in groups that makes sense to them. Card sorting also allows for blank cards to be given to users so they can add in concepts they feel are missing. We led our subcommittee through a card-sort activity, acting as various user groups of the hub, to highlight how different people would organize and use information differently. The results from the card sort allowed us to create several potential test sites.

Additionally, we videotaped users completing several tasks with iterations of the portal. For these tests, we utilized the hub production site and developed two sandbox sites (sandbox A and sandbox B) that were used for the various searching activities (find information about your program, find information about researchers working in a particular area, locate funding opportunities, and find a definition of "translational research"). Each of the three sites had different elements highlighted that we identified through the card-sort process.

The production site had numerous and diverse top-level menu items (About, For Researchers, For the Public, Training, Resources, Feedback, and Support) and no consistent landing pages (a landing page is the main page you'd arrive at after you clicked on any top-level menu items). Sandbox A was organized around three role-based menus (About, Research, and Community) and utilized landing pages with a list of navigable links. Sandbox B was organized around three action-based menus (About, Find Resources, and Find People) and featured landing pages with two levels of tabs.

We summarized and analyzed the results from our various volunteers and quantified their individual comments (e.g., drop-down menus highly preferred; don't want to navigate through menus but would rather get directly to the information desired; menu items too ambiguous). One of the most interesting findings was that users did not utilize menus to navigate the site but went straight for the search box (maybe not such a surprise!). Despite user preference for searching over menu-guided navigation, the search functionality was not optimal. Feedback indicated that many users found the search results too complex and expressed a desire for a tool that would facilitate a simple search of the hub content. As this echoed a discussion we had had earlier within the larger hub committee, we were happy to see that our librarian understanding of users' needs meshed with our volunteers' experience.

Based on the group's expertise and the input from the test subjects in the card-sort/task finding we wrote up our recommendations and submitted the report to the

CTSI administration.[2] These included disambiguating terms used on the front page (e.g., Cores/Programs; Help/Support), facilitating access or account creation, improving search functionality to allow for an Advanced Search within specific content areas, and reducing the amount of content on the portal's front page.

Once the redesign project was completed, the hub committee disbanded. Through our participation, we had made valuable connections with others involved in the support of the Indiana CTSI. Several months later, I was asked to join the CTSI Communications Work Group, the advisory group for public relations efforts including the Indiana CTSI newsletter. The committee's role was to discuss the myriad research projects being conducted by Indiana CTSI-funded researchers to determine if any of these projects would make suitable stories for the newsletter. While I wasn't usually the one reporting on research projects or bringing ideas to the table for stories, this was a great way to learn about various projects going on within the CTSI, and this helped me identify possible collaborations. I also provided an editorial eye for the newsletter before it went out. There was usually a quick turnaround between reviewing the newsletter and when it was sent out via e-mail, and I know that my contributions helped to bring both clarity and a consistent internal style to the newsletter.

As I previously mentioned, participating in these local committees and work groups was an immense help in making connections and developing productive relationships with people within the CTSI and across our institution. For instance, through the Communications Work Group, I worked closely with the person in charge of the newsletter, who also worked on communications for the medical school. Developing this relationship ensured a channel to having library events, activities, and classes more widely publicized within IUSM. Additionally, since they'd come to value our expertise, CTSI administration would occasionally contact the medical librarians for assistance. Common questions included copyright issues, locating psychological tests and instruments, peer review of planning documents, and locating standardized codes for medical devices.

EVALUATION AND TRACKING PROGRAM

The other main project area in which I've been heavily involved is on the CTSI's Evaluation and Tracking Program. I have worked closely with our local CTSI program and have also participated nationally as a member of the evaluation key function committee (KFC) and chair of an evaluation working group.

My initial involvement—and much of my current involvement—with the Evaluation and Tracking Program at our CTSI came about through bibliometrics. Bibliometrics is the quantitative analysis of publications and often the focus is analyzing citations to papers and quantifying that information. Some resources that provide bibliometric information (such as citing articles, h-index, journal information, author affiliation/department, and index terms) include Scopus, Web of Science, and

Google Scholar. In my role, using bibliometrics involves tracking journals in which our CTSI researchers publish, as well as identifying their coauthors, collaborators, and partners both within and outside their home universities. We were interested in setting a baseline for where and with whom our researchers publish and seeing if their collaborations change over time. Additionally, we are interested in which programs within the CTSI are being utilized and cited in the articles, which may help determine programs that are being heavily used as well as those that need to be better publicized. I have presented on my work at our annual CTSI meeting and have copublished an article on the use of social-networking tools in using publication data to demonstrate the concentrations of research areas within our CTSI.[3]

My work with my local evaluation program colleagues led me to begin attending monthly conference calls for the evaluation KFC and to interact more with Clinical and Translational Science Award (CTSA) evaluators from across the country. At first I felt very out of place as I'm not a full-time evaluator, but when the group discussed difficulties in getting researchers to cite the CTSA grant in publications and various options used at different institutions to attempt to track researcher collaborations, I was able to contribute to these conversations. Additionally, acronyms such as KFC (key function committee), NCRR (National Center for Research Resources), NCATS (National Center for Advancing Translational Sciences), and NOGA (notice of grant award) now have meaning to me and I'm able to understand them, use them, and not have to Google every acronym when I'm on a conference call.

As I gained experience with this group, I progressed from participating on the calls to working with a national CTSA definitions work group charged with defining "publication" for CTSA reporting purposes. This was important because CTSA institutions are required to submit an annual progress report (APR) to the National Institutes of Health (NIH), including a list of publications that derived from CTSA grant funding. CTSA institutions have struggled with how to uniformly define publications, and while this initially seemed very straightforward, the project quickly took on a life of its own. Some issues included the following: Is a publication only a journal article, book chapter, or monograph? Does it have to be peer reviewed? Do posters, blogs, or websites count? What percentage of someone's time needs to be related to a publication for it to "count" as being funded by a CTSA? Coming up with a succinct but comprehensive and overarching definition of "publication" regarding CTSAs and NIH reporting requirements took many months, numerous conference calls, and multiple iterations of the final document. Finally our national work group put forward our recommended definition to the evaluation KFC. The definition was accepted, which means that for reporting, all CTSAs should be using the same agreed-upon definition for reporting CTSA publications to NIH.

Through my work with the evaluation KFC, I also became more involved with its bibliometrics working group (BWG) and was asked to serve as cochair. The BWG's purpose was to determine what metrics are used by individual CTSAs in evaluation reporting; how bibliometrics are used across different fields; and how to do this analysis beyond medical research efforts. If I accepted this position, I would be required to be chair of the BWG the following year. While I was already doing everything that would be required of a cochair—namely, attending conference calls and participating in the discussions—being chair would involve significantly more responsibilities. In addition to running the monthly conference calls, communicating with the administrative support assigned to our group, and reminding people of what they had agreed to do, I'd also have to stay on top of broader discussions within the evaluation KFC and bring any relevant concerns to the BWG. While anyone could attend both the evaluation KFC and BWG conference calls, many people are involved in multiple aspects of their CTSAs and trying to keep on top of everything and attending every meeting becomes difficult.

Accepting this position was a scary proposition. While many BWG members were full-time evaluators, I didn't (and still don't) view myself as an evaluator, and I didn't know if I had the necessary background, skills, and expertise to take on this role. But there was a definite need, I was already attending the calls, and I realized this really was a great opportunity to learn about something new and challenge myself in a new role. So I agreed. Taking on this new role was uncomfortable and scary at first, but when we start talking about tracking publications, ways to encourage researchers to cite their institution's CTSA grant number, how to support NIH public access policy compliance, and so forth, I felt at home. Librarians are already doing many of these things: We already compile data about publications, and we're frequently trying to create compelling stories about the impact of our work (or in this case, researchers' research projects). Not only are we already doing these types of things, but also we often have a better grasp of the information tools that exist, their benefits and shortfalls, and the need to check in more than one place, as everything is *not* in PubMed (or in Google, for that matter). In short, this work can be a perfect fit for librarians! It was also a bit of a relief to know that there were other librarians on the BWG and not just full-time evaluators; I felt more comfortable knowing that some of my own tribe were present too. As far as I know, I was the first librarian to chair a national CTSA working group, and it may be a coincidence, but the next two chairs of the BWG also happened to be librarians.

The biggest project I worked on while cochair/chair of the BWG was a survey that was being sent out to all CTSA institutions mainly focused on publications and reporting requirements. This survey project preceded my involvement with the BWG, but it had never come to fruition. The first step was to develop and refine the survey's questions. Questions included the data sources CTSAs used to find grant-related publications; local response rates; the number of publications claimed (with PubMed Central identifiers or PMCIDs); the number of publications CTSAs wanted to claim but couldn't because they were not in compliance with the NIH public access policy; the types of people involved in collecting publication information; the frequency of data collection; and difficulties in collecting the data. Additionally, we asked questions to help expose contexts for publication data (in other words, what kinds of stories do people want to tell that demonstrate impact or give their CTSA-funded publications other meaning). While there were discussions on the BWG conference calls about these questions, for the most part, the work to final-ize the survey was done by two other people (at two different institutions) and me. In addition to determining exactly how the questions should be worded, we worked out the logistics, including what tool to use to administer the survey, who was the ideal target audience for the survey, and our plans to analyze and report the response data. While this may seem outside of the "normal" librarian role, and I didn't ever envision myself doing this, as librarians, we definitely have the skills and expertise to help design these sorts of surveys.

The experience of completing this survey also gave me a new understanding of administrative burden. Specifically, I gained firsthand experience with seemingly over-the-top reporting requirements. After a lot of work to finalize the survey and decide the most appropriate target audience (e.g., the administration KFC or a group for CTSA administrators), we had to get the survey approved before it could be dis-tributed. Ironically, this required us to fill out a survey detailing what we were asking in our survey, identifying the target audience, explaining the importance of doing this particular survey, describing what we would do with the results, and so forth. While I understand the intent (to help avoid surveying people to death with poorly designed questionnaires), filling out the survey about the survey took forty minutes; then there was a delay while our survey was approved. Finally, it was approved and we were able to move forward with distribution.

This step gave me an opportunity to leverage another skill I use in my daily work: getting people to respond to e-mails, requests, surveys, and so forth. This is an ongo-ing challenge for many people, whether it's for work or personal communications. Some of the tricks I've learned to be successful in getting useful responses include the following: be clear about the respondents' role/responsibility (don't make them guess, as they may either not respond or not give you useful responses); tell them what information they will need to have on hand before starting the survey (don't make them stop the survey to look for something as they may not come back); give a clear deadline; and follow up with either the group or individuals who need to respond. Generally speaking, I know that it helps me to have clear expectations laid out when I'm asked for information, and this helps me prioritize my work, so I try to do the same when making requests of others. Our survey had a 70 percent response rate, which we thought was more than adequate.

The purpose of this particular survey was to identify methods used to report publications, how the data is used for strategic planning, any difficulties in col-lecting publication data, and how the data is used to the show impact. We found out that the methods for identifying and reporting publications data were different among pilot funding recipients, trainees, and those using a CTSA core or service; the most common collection method was using a "validated" subset of publica-tions in conjunction with manual analysis and curation. Examples of validated data sources include PubMed/MEDLINE, NIH RePORTER, Elsevier Scopus/SciVal, and institutional repositories/administrative databases. The most common ways in which publication data is being used for strategic planning include increasing outreach around acknowledging the CTSA in publications; identifying strengths of our CTSA; justifying institution-contributed funds; and increasing outreach/ support around NIH public access policy. Difficulties in collecting publication data include lack of reporting from investigators; forgetting to cite CTSA programs; delay between receiving support and actual publication; manual validation being time consuming and complicated; and confusion about which CTSA programs to cite. On a more positive note, data is being used to demonstrate impact through the breadth of research endeavors at an institution; highlighting new discoveries; new collaborations emerging within (and across) institutions; and showcasing benefits of a CTSA to a given institution.

One challenge that came up in the survey, and that CTSAs are still struggling with, is how to demonstrate the impact of our researchers' work based on their publications. Numbers can be a starting point, but we are increasingly seeing the need to paint a picture, tell a story, or otherwise provide context for the numbers or metrics we are reporting. This can be incredibly hard, especially when something that appears as simple as "report the number of publications from your CTSA" turns out to mean very different things to different people at different CTSA institutions.

OUTCOMES

One of the great things about being involved with a project such as this, aside from the end result of actually seeing it come to fruition, is the chance to share your findings. After we analyzed the survey results, we created a poster for the annual face-to-face meeting of the evaluation KFC. We were also asked to present the findings briefly during the meeting as part of the scheduled program. As it happened, the administration KFC was holding their face-to-face meeting the next day and wanted us to present the findings there too. In the end, we were able to create three scholarly products out of the survey, which is always a nice validation for all the work and time that went into making the survey a reality.

Finally, as BWG chair, I was responsible for planning work group activities. I had to submit an annual report to update the status of ongoing projects, as well as defining projects we intended to work on for the upcoming year. For any new projects, I had to describe how they would align with the strategic goals of the CTSAs, explain the deliverables coming out of these projects, and state the time frame to accomplish these various projects. One example of a new BWG project arose from attending the evaluation KFC face-to-face meeting. At this meeting, participants agreed on a series of clinical metrics that were of the most importance to the evaluation KFC. Three of the clinical metrics dealt with publications, and it fell to the BWG to tackle how to establish these metrics: time to publication; influence of research publications; and time of publication to research synthesis. I sought volunteers within the BWG to form small groups to begin work on these. As it turned out, each group was headed up by a librarian. We began to lead our respective groups to think through each of these metrics and to discuss how these were regarded, viewed, and practiced at our various institutions. For reasons I'll discuss later, the BWG was disbanded and the project called off before we could complete our work.

FUTURE PLANS

I am currently involved in two CTSA/CTSI projects. The first is a publication classification project, led by New York University's (NYU) CTSA, with input and collaboration from various CTSAs across the country, including our CTSI. NYU is building a publication classifier, a program that would automatically categorize articles into the respective translational levels based on title and abstract. The idea is that one could input a set of PubMed identifiers (PMIDs) and the classifier would determine which articles fell into T0, T1, T2, T3, or T4 (basic science, clinical research, clinical practice, or policy) categories. Ultimately, this tool could help to efficiently highlight the relationship between CTSA grant funding and different areas of translational research.

Determining the criteria for each of these "T" categories has been an interesting effort, and much time has been spent defining the rules for each of these categories. We have done several iterations of using these classification rules with actual CTSA-funded articles. Alisa Surkis, translational librarian at NYU, has been doing the lion's share of continuing to move this project forward and refining rules so that they can be applied consistently (for more information, see chapter 17). I contribute to this project by working with our associate director of evaluation and tracking to individually review abstracts, compare our results and talk about our discrepancies, and to then compare our results with the larger national group. This is still a work in progress (the classifier is still being developed), but this publication classification tool has been an interesting project, and I look forward to continuing my contribution.

My other current CTSA project is also a team effort with the associate director (AD) of evaluation and tracking here at the Indiana CTSI. The AD oversees all of the evaluating and tracking for the CTSA, including coordinating all the evaluation reporting for all the programs of the CTSI. My role and work focuses on the bibliometrics aspects of reporting. As previously mentioned I've worked on tracking and documenting CTSI publications to show publication patterns among our CTSI researchers for many years now. As an extension of my support for our researchers for compliance with the NIH public access policy, I have recently been added as a delegate in My NCBI for the primary investigator (PI) of the Indiana CTSI to help track, monitor, and achieve compliance for all articles that are citing our CTSI-funded research. Additionally, whenever a researcher receives funds from our CTSI, my contact information is provided in their award letter. The intent is to give them a contact to help with acquiring a PMCID for any publications that will result from the CTSI funding. In addition to benefiting researchers, who often have questions about compliance, this benefits the CTSI, as only publications that cite the CTSI grant and have a PMCID can be "counted" as related publications in the annual report. This can be a complicated process, in part because our CTSA has researchers at three different universities across the state, but I have contacts at all universities to aid in the compliance process. I've also created protocols, handouts, and sample letters for compliance that are available on our library web page. We plan to add this information to the CTSI Hub as well.

CHALLENGES

Developing and maintaining relationships is always hard, and in a new environment with no defined parameters, it can be even more difficult. Even though our efforts to integrate with the CTSI were supported from library administration from the beginning, there was never an overarching plan or clear way forward for the library's involvement with the CTSI. Some of us were able to initially get our foot in the door, but it can be hard to maintain those relationships without sustained support. This may be why most of my "success" stories stem from personal connections/interactions and a willingness to step out of my comfort zone and try new things.

Additionally, there have been changes within the CTSA program over the years. Initially the CTSA fell under the NCRR (National Center for Research Resources) at NIH, but over time, as the CTSA program grew, it eventually left the NCRR and morphed into a distinct NIH center, the NCATS. This change caused a lot of uncertainty in moving forward with the KFCs and ultimately resulted in dramatic changes in infrastructure; in fact, the KFCs and their subgroups, like the BWG, don't exist anymore. Many of the conference calls leading up to the transition from NCRR to NCATS featured discussions about the value of the evaluation KFC, how to demonstrate its value to NIH, and determining next steps for CTSA evaluators if the KFC structure was dismantled. Unfortunately, the changes did impact the evaluation KFC and its subgroups, and we lost our collaborative framework for evaluation metrics. This also affected several projects, including the development of metrics related to publications described above. I believe the fact that the KFC and BWG no longer exist are as a consequence of NIH changes beyond our control and in no way a reflection on the value or quality of the group's work. The changing nature of the larger CTSA program is an ongoing challenge, and it can be disheartening to spend a lot of time on a project and not be able to see it through to completion.

LESSONS LEARNED

I've sprinkled in some lessons learned throughout this case study, but I've also collected them here:

- Be willing to take risks. This is probably not surprising, but hopefully serves as a good reminder. I was lucky in that I was invited to sit at the table and go to meetings at the beginning, but maintaining those relationships and volunteering to take on responsibilities when it may be out of your comfort zone is a great way to develop new skills and gain some confidence in your current abilities.
- Things might not work—and that's okay! I initially worked on a project with one of the CTSI programs, I met with a lot of people, and then nothing came of it. In hindsight, I think what I was asked to do wasn't the best for my skill set, I didn't have the tools/authority to accomplish it, and the project fizzled. It happens. And I survived.
- It's okay to listen and not speak up, right away anyway. I'm an extrovert, so it may be easier for me to voice my opinion than it is for more introverted people, but know that it's generally okay (unless you're the main speaker) to just listen, take in everything you can, observe body language, and figure out who would be a likely champion or collaborator. Sometimes, you may feel that someone else in your library would be better suited to partner with a particular group. At the very least, you can bring back information to your library colleagues about the activities of your institution or issues at the national CTSA level. You can also take notes on things that you can follow up on with people if you don't want to speak up in the moment.
- Remember that you're in the room for a reason. Assume that people think you have something to offer and that at least one person in the room or on the conference call likes you, respects your value, and doesn't think you're an idiot, and go with that. Have faith in people and be confident that you and your expertise *are* valuable to the people in the room (even if they don't always acknowledge it).
- Support from library administration makes things easier but isn't an absolute requirement. During the tenure of our CTSI, our library director retired and our library was director-less for a while. Our work with the CTSI still continued.
- Be nice to people. This is a more general life rule, but I think being nice, respectful, and genuinely interested in others can go a long way in making people be more willing to work with you.
- Partner, partner, partner! You never know when the contact you make will result in a great relationship that can be mutually beneficial. Also, you always learn something new or gain a different perspective.
- Many of the varied skills and expertise we have as librarians can be used in numerous facets or areas of translational research. I happened to work more on the evaluation and publications side, but I know several librarian colleagues who are involved with the biomedical informatics, community engagement, and training programs of their CTSAs.
- Share what you learn at CTSA meetings (outside of the library) with those inside the library. It can be helpful for your colleagues to understand the work you do and how the library's and librarians' visibility is raised by your work.

At the risk of stating the obvious, roles for librarians are constantly changing. It is exciting to see and experience how our skills can be used in many different aspects of the translational research enterprise. Being willing to take risks (and even fail sometimes), talk to people outside of our libraries, and speak up even when we're not quite sure how we will fit can lead to interesting collaborations that highlight the skills we already possess in new ways.

NOTES

1. Indiana University. What is the Indiana CTSI Hub, and how do I register for an account? https://kb.iu.edu/d/bafv. Accessed January 8, 2015.

2. Davis B, Hardwick E, Odell JD, Skopelja EN, Shankar A, Whipple EC. CTSA hub usability report. http://hdl.handle.net/1805/5758. Accessed January 30, 2015.

3. Hunt JD, Whipple EC, McGowan JJ. Use of social network analysis tools to validate a resources infrastructure for interinstitutional translational research: A case study. *J Med Libr Assoc.* 2012 Jan;100(1):48–54.

17

Assessing Impact through Publications

Metrics That Tell a Story

Alisa Surkis

INTRODUCTION

The New York University (NYU) School of Medicine received a Clinical and Translational Science Award (CTSA) in 2009 in partnership with other NYU schools, including the colleges of dentistry and nursing, the School of Engineering, and nine of the public hospitals that are part of the Health and Hospitals Corporation (HHC) of New York City. The NYU-HHC Clinical and Translational Science Institute (CTSI) funded by this grant has two co-principal investigators (PIs): Dr. Bruce Cronstein, a translational researcher, and Dr. Judith Hochman, a clinical researcher.

In response to the formation of the NYU-HHC CTSI, the NYU Health Sciences Library (NYUHSL) created a new translational science librarian position in 2010, and I started in this position in January of 2011 as a new librarian. Prior to making the career change to librarianship, I had done my doctoral work in experimental and computational neuroscience and then worked for more than ten years writing software to collect and analyze data and model visual systems for vision science researchers. I enjoyed working in support of research, problem-solving programming, and dealing with the organization of data and information. In my shift to librarianship, I hoped to incorporate these same elements but to broaden the scope of the challenges I would face and, with that, the possible solutions. I was fortunate to find a position with a wide-ranging set of responsibilities and the latitude to approach these creatively.

There was no road map for library support of and integration with the fairly new CTSI for a new librarian in a new position. I read up on the CTSA program in general and the NYU-HHC CTSI in particular, as well as seeking out the fairly sparse literature at the time on what other librarians were doing in support of CTSA programs. I was asked to introduce myself at a CTSI executive committee meeting, and I asked if I could sit in on these meetings regularly; this was, by far, the most important step I took in figuring out my new role. Sitting in on those meetings each month allowed me to gain insight into the needs of the program and allowed the attendees from across the institution to get to know me; it also meant I was there when someone thought to say, "Oh, can the library help with that?"

The initial roles I took on, and so the types of support the CTSI looked to me to provide, were centered on publications. The first task that came my way was maintaining National Institutes of Health (NIH) public access policy compliance for CTSI publications, a very natural thing to ask of the librarian at the table. Another reasonable request to make of a librarian is assistance with publication tracking; as this is also a core task for program evaluation, I was invited to join the CTSI's evaluation working group.

I will describe in detail two projects that I have been involved with, one as part of my work on the CTSI's evaluation working group and one that grew out of my role on the national evaluation key function committee's (KFC) bibliometrics work group. Both projects share the goal of developing publication metrics that tell a more complete or relevant story about the impact of a CTSI than the default metrics, such as the numbers of publications acknowledging a CTSA grant or the impact factors of those publication's journals. The first project involved finding a way to produce a more nuanced picture of the publication output of our CTSI through introducing the concepts of direct and indirect benefit into publication tracking. The project that grew out of the bibliometrics work group involves developing a machine-learning approach to classifying publications along the translational research spectrum.

PUBLICATION TRACKING

The evaluation working group was formed out of need. The NYU-HHC CTSI had less than one full-time equivalent dedicated to evaluation, so help was enlisted from across the organization. The working group was led by the director of evaluation and manned by representatives from the CTSI's administration and from each of the cores (e.g., biostatistics and informatics). One of the core functions of the evaluation working group was tracking publications; that is, identifying research papers that had benefited from the CTSI in some way, such as receiving a pilot projects award or using the CTSI's Clinical Research Center. Tracking publications is important for grant administration because it is generally seen as a key marker of success.

When I joined the CTSI, the only publications being tracked were those that cited the CTSI grant number. This was problematic for two reasons: first, it can be difficult to ensure investigators cite the grant appropriately, so I knew these publications represented only a subset of all articles that utilized CTSI resources. Additionally, I quickly realized through my participation in the bibliometrics work group that there was a wide variation in how different CTSA institutions counted their publications. By only counting publications linked directly to the CTSA grant number, we were at one end of the spectrum and in the minority. At the other end of the spectrum were institutions that counted all publications by all researchers who had used any CTSA services. This creates a problem in that institutions that track only those publications that claim direct support may appear to be less "productive" than those that track all publications that utilized CTSA resources or services. And neither of these numbers reveals much, if anything, about the impact of the CTSA, which should be the overarching goal of program evaluation. I began to develop a solution that would address both problems—it would allow our CTSI to accurately and efficiently track all publications associated with our CTSA funding and would also help to answer questions about impact.

Tracking only publications that cite a CTSA grant number is easily done; a quick search of a grant number in PubMed will retrieve most, if not all, of the publications in question. This method, however, results in a significant undercounting of the publications that benefit from CTSI support, since many investigators who receive support fail to acknowledge the CTSA grant in their publication. Tracking all publications from all researchers who had interacted with the CTSI would be more time consuming, though I could take advantage of a bibliography of faculty publications NYUHSL has maintained for many years.[1] This count of publications, though, would be a significant overrepresentation since CTSA support for one project does not mean that all of an investigator's projects utilized or benefited from the CTSA.

Developing any type of publication tracking between these two extremes would require greater effort but would also be a more accurate reflection of the true output of the CTSI. In developing this middle-ground methodology, I decided that a two-tiered approach of identifying publications would simultaneously increase publication counts and accuracy while also providing a clearer picture of the impact of the CTSI.

My idea was that a construct of direct versus indirect benefit would help illuminate the immediate (direct) versus downstream (indirect) effects of the CTSI. This construct would help demonstrate how the effects of the CTSI propagate through the research process to better illustrate the complex impact of our CTSI. The basic definitions of these levels of benefit are that a study is said to receive direct benefit when it uses CTSI funding, goods, or services, and a study is said to receive indirect benefit when it uses CTSI facilities (e.g., use of the CTSI's Clinical Research Center that is paid for off of the investigator's grant) or when the study makes use of results of another study that received direct benefit from the CTSI (e.g., line of research based on the initial project or review article including results of project).

For several years, I did this process manually. I made use of the library's faculty bibliography, which includes faculty from the medical school and the colleges of dentistry and nursing. Having these publication lists available meant that I could bypass searching multiple databases to identify faculty publications. It also obviated the need to dig into whether the publications my search returned were from the investigator I was interested in or were authored by another, similarly named investigator (i.e., resolving name disambiguation). For faculty from other NYU schools or HHC investigators, I searched in PubMed and Web of Science.

CTSI administrative personnel provided me with data on CTSI-supported projects. For some projects this included an abstract; for others, just a project title. Any publication that acknowledged the CTSA grant was assumed to have directly benefited from the CTSI. For other publications, I compared the title and abstract of the publication to whatever information I had on the investigator's CTSI supported projects. If the publication appeared to describe the supported project, I would count that publication in the direct benefit category. If the publication described a project that built on the CTSI supported project, used a method developed with CTSI support, or included the CTSI-supported project in a review, I would count it in the indirect benefit category.

Ultimately, this approach of tracking both direct and indirect publications was adopted by the NYU-HHC CTSI. It has been used for progress reports, advisory board presentations, and the 2015 CTSA application. However, this process was time consuming and certainly contained a degree of error as it relied on my judgment as to how a publication related to a project listed.

As one of my objectives was to increase the efficiency of publication tracking, I experimented with various approaches to automate some part of the process or spread the workload among more people. For example, I built a shared Mendeley library and set up workflows so that people from across a number of CTSI programs could directly input relevant publications, but between personnel changes and competing demands on people's time, that system broke down. The NYU-HHC CTSI uses WebCAMP, a tracking program developed at Cornell and used by a number of CTSA institutions, and I explored the use of one of the WebCAMP modules to reach out to investigators to query them about their publications. Ultimately I concluded that this would not work without customization of that system, and we did not have the resources for that.

Finally in 2014, while preparing for the renewal application for our CTSA grant, I worked with both administration and evaluation people in the CTSI to begin to automate some aspects of the process of collecting relevant publications. CTSI administrative personnel used WebCAMP to generate and export a list of investigator names, projects, and dates of service. I wrote a program in Matlab to query the library's faculty bibliography API (application program interface)[1] for articles published after the date of service and to output these publications to a spreadsheet. Evaluation personnel in the CTSI created a survey using Qualtrics that was sent out to all investigators who had received either pilot awards from the CTSI or support through one of the CTSI's resource-allocation programs. The survey asked, for each publication, whether it had directly or indirectly benefited (as defined in the survey) from CTSI services. Figure 17.1 shows a graph of direct and indirect publications for one of the CTSI's resource-allocation programs.

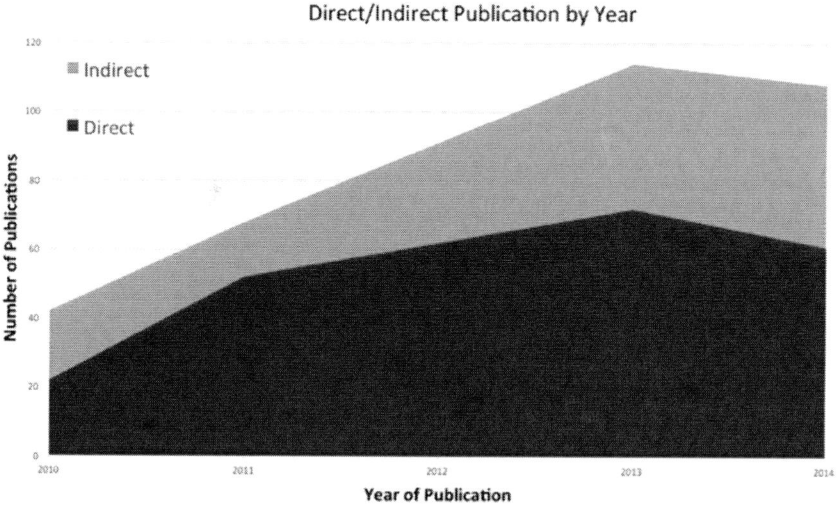

Direct/Indirect Publication by Year

Figure 17.1. Number of direct and indirect publications by year was used as a way to capture the downstream effects of CTSI support.

The survey was only sent out once due to time constraints, but the response rate was almost 40 percent. Responses identified a number of publications as indirectly benefiting from CTSI support that I had not previously attributed to the CTSI, which helps us more accurately track CTSI support of projects. I am currently working with administration and evaluation personnel to streamline this workflow to make use of the automated elements that were developed and track responses. Additionally, I will modify my Matlab code so that investigators are not queried multiple times about the same publications. While this is not a perfect solution to the publication tracking problem, it increases the accuracy of our reporting, reduces the manual elements of the process, and can be done with the personnel and resources at hand.

PUBLICATION CLASSIFICATION

Project Initiation

Before it was disbanded by the National Center for Advancing Translational Sciences (NCATS) in 2014, the national consortium of CTSA programs had an extensive infrastructure of KFCs, including one for evaluation, and related work groups. One of the evaluation KFC work groups was the bibliometrics work group. I served as the cochair of that group from the fall of 2013 until the consortium was disbanded in the winter of 2014.

In 2013, the evaluation KFC was engaged in a project to create operational definitions for a set of common metrics for the CTSA programs. A set of fifteen common metrics had been identified,[2] and relevant work groups were tasked with defining a number of measurement attributes, including a description of the metric, the rationale for it, and the data sources. The bibliometrics work group was tasked with defining the three publication-related metrics: time to publication, influence of a research publication, and time from publication to research synthesis.

As bibliometrics cochair, I led the group addressing the influence of a research publication, but the consortium was disbanded by NCATS before we made meaningful progress on that metric. However, in considering the concept of research publication influence, I arrived at an idea for a metric that I thought could address the CTSA mission more directly than existing publication metrics. Citation counts—the number of times a publication is cited in other articles—may speak to impact but provide no information on where that impact is seen or felt. For example, a publication could have a large citation count, but if those citations all come from publications within the same field, that would indicate a narrow sphere of influence.

Since the goal of the CTSA program is to move discoveries from the bench to the bedside into the community, I wanted a metric that could capture knowledge translation; that is, whether a publication was influencing work in other areas along the translational research spectrum. This metric would have to compare the categorization of an article along the translational research spectrum to the categorizations of that article's citations. While this could be a valuable way to demonstrate the impact of a publication on translational research, manual categorization of articles is too time consuming to make this feasible. Therefore, the first step toward developing a knowledge translational metric would be to see if a machine-learning approach can successfully categorize articles along the translational research spectrum.

Machine Learning

There are a number of methods for automated text classification. The basic idea behind each is that a classifier is built by compiling a training set and using this to "teach" an algorithm, which features the text in question associated with a given category (see figure 17.2).

In this case, the text would be a publication. The features are words, most commonly from the title or abstract of a publication, but can also be sets of words, such as journal titles or extracted concepts, including medical subject headings (MeSH).

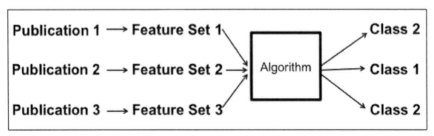

Figure 17.2. Each publication is represented by a set of features (e.g., words in title and abstract), and each feature set is associated with a given class (e.g., T0 and not T0).

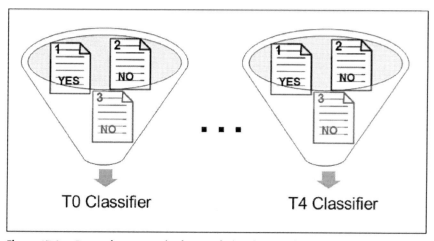

Figure 17.3. For each category in the translational research spectrum, the training set consists of publications, represented by a set of features, and whether manual coding has placed them in a given category.

A training set is assembled and a classifier built for each category along the translational spectrum by manually labeling each publication as either positive or negative for each category (see figure 17.3). The algorithm then "learns" which features of the publications associate most strongly with each category.

While this seems clear cut in theory, it is not always possible to arrive at an algorithm that will perform well in classifying text. In order to build a classifier with good performance, there must exist features of the publications in a given category that distinguish them from publications that are not in that category. For example, if most articles in the category T2 have the words "clinical" and "trial" somewhere in the title or abstract, and most articles that do not fall within T2 do not have those words in the title or abstract, then the algorithm would learn that those words were important in classifying an article as T2, and the classifier would be able to perform well. This project would test whether the publications that fell within a particular category were distinct enough to produce a classifier that performed well.

Assembling a Team

I was familiar with the basic concepts behind machine learning and knew that there were informaticians at our Center for Health Informatics and Bioinformatics (CHIBI) who had expertise in the area of text classification. I approached Laurence Fu about this project, and it sufficiently aligned with his interests, so he agreed to collaborate. However, early in the project, he took a position in industry, and we were fortunate to gain Yindalon Aphinyanaphongs, another text classification expert in CHIBI, as a collaborator.

I hoped to find other collaborators in the bibliometrics work group and described my idea both to the group I was leading on defining the influence of a research publication and to the broader bibliometrics work group. While there was no expressed interest in this specific project, on one of the bibliometrics work group calls, Jan Hogle, the associate director for evaluation at the University of Wisconsin Institute for Clinical and Translational Research (ICTR), described the work her group was doing in manually classifying publications along the translational spectrum.

I saw an opportunity and reached out to Hogle to ask if I could use the coding she had done as part of the training set for my project. This was a fortunate development: Hogle had been the chair of the definitions work group within the evaluation KFC, and in speaking with her, I realized that I had glossed over the issue of what categories of translational research to use and how to define them. This lack of definition would present a major hurdle in assembling a training set. Fortunately, Hogle not only agreed to collaborate on the project but also brought in several additional collaborators from Wisconsin who assisted at various points in the project: Trisha Adamus, the data, network, and translational librarian; Kate Westaby, an evaluation research specialist; and Alexis Tavano, a coordinator for the collaboration of the Wisconsin ICTR with the Marshfield clinic.

Additionally, as Hogle had been more involved in the CTSA consortium than I had, and had a broader network, she was able to bring in collaborators from three additional institutions: Indiana University (IU), Medical College of Wisconsin (MCW), and Virginia Commonwealth University (VCU). These collaborators are as follows: Joe Hunt, associate director of the tracking and evaluation program, and Beth Whipple, research informationist/assistant librarian, from the IU CTSI; Emily Connors, evaluator for the MCW CTSI, and later replaced in her position at MCW and on the project by Meridith Mueller; and Paul Mazmanian, director of the evaluation core, and Deborah DiazGranados, program evaluator for the VCU Center for Clinical and Translational Research (CCTR).

Establishing the collaboration with Hogle was key to this project. In addition to her depth of experience in dealing with definitions around translational research, her connections led to a project team that spanned five CTSA programs. This breadth of participation brought a broader perspective on the definitions, more hands to do the manual coding, and more use cases to inform the project. Also, agreement on definitions across a larger number of CTSAs would be more likely to influence other CTSAs to adopt those definitions and so be able to make use of the classifiers.

Agreeing on Definitions

The starting point for the categories along the translational spectrum and their definitions was the Institute of Medicine CTSA report.[3] This report defined five stages of translational research and served as the starting point for the more detailed definitions that had been developed at Wisconsin, which also drew on the Harvard Catalyst definitions.[4] At MCW they had been using six categories that drew on the definitions from Wisconsin and Harvard, as well as from several other sources.[5-8] VCU had been using the definitions from the 2012 article by Blumberg and colleagues,[9] with that article having served as a basis for the Institute of Medicine (IOM) definitions. All of these sets of definitions were fairly similar, so despite a few sticking points along the way, it was a fairly smooth process to come to a set of definitions for categories from T0 to T4 that all the collaborators were willing to use.

Testing the Definitions

It became clear that agreeing on definitions was only a first step. In order to test our understanding of the definitions, I assembled a pilot set of publications to be classified by all the collaborating institutions. My initial approach was to seek out publications that would be particularly difficult to categorize in order to determine where our common understanding of the definitions broke down. The group at Wisconsin provided a set of thirty-two publications that they had had difficulty categorizing, and I distributed these to the group of ten collaborators from five institutions. When I received the coding of the test set back, I found that our shared understanding of the definitions broke down everywhere; there was not one publication on which everyone agreed as to the category.

This led to a second pilot with a new approach. I wrote a program in Matlab to call the NCBI programming utilities to search for all publications that were indexed to any of our five CTSA grants and then randomly select five publications from each institution. This was a small-scale version of the planned approach for assembling the full training set, so the assumption was that this approach would give a more accurate reflection of the agreement, or lack of agreement, we might encounter in building the training set.

The results of the second pilot project were better, though not encouraging. Agreement across all coders was reached on only five of the twenty-five publications. In addition to this training set, we also revisited eleven of the publications from the initial pilot to see if the discussion of those articles had impacted their coding. There was still not consensus on any of those eleven articles, although the coding had converged to some degree. Taking both sets into account, we had agreement on 14 percent of the publications, with an additional 11 percent on which all but one coder agreed.

While the second exercise had a slightly better outcome than the first, the wide variation in interpretations of the definitions did not bode well for the prospect of assembling a training set. I was aware that checklists were used to improve the consistency in measures of clinical performance across assessors,[10,11] so I proposed that we take a similar approach as a way to improve the consistency of our coding (inter-rater reliability). I drafted a checklist for each of the categories, and we went through several rounds of input and editing to arrive at a checklist that the group agreed to use. For each category of translational research, there were between four and twelve questions; if a coder answered yes to any question, they would put the article in that category.

256   *Alisa Surkis*

Table 17.1. Examples of checklist items used to improve the consistency of coding

T0 core definition: BASIC BIOMEDICAL RESEARCH
Identification of opportunities and approaches to health problems

| Checklist example 1 | Does the research involve study of mechanisms, relationships, or modification of proteins, DNA, or cells? |
| Checklist example 2 | Does the research explore a biological, social, or behavioral mechanism, including the mechanism underlying the presence or progression of a disease? |

T3 core definition: TRANSLATION TO PRACTICE
Practice guidelines to health practices

| Checklist example 1 | Does the research study inconsistency or variation in the application of a diagnosis or intervention? |
| Checklist example 2 | Does the research identify problems with effective health-care delivery in practice or community settings? |

The group used the new checklist to revisit the thirty-six articles, not only to categorize the publications but also to record which checklist items led to that categorization. This round of coding produced consensus on 31 percent of the articles, up from 14 percent. All but one coder agreed on an additional 36 percent of publications, up from 11 percent. This was a marked improvement, and because of the inclusion of the checklist items, it was now clear as to how each person had arrived at the determination of which category to assign to a publication. Table 17.1 shows some examples of checklist items.

Current Status and Next Steps

It was decided that with the checklist approach, it was now time to assemble the full training set. We have assembled the training set and run a preliminary analysis. The results are very encouraging. Performance of a classifier is measured by plotting the number of true positives—publications that the classifier correctly classified—versus the number of false positives—publications incorrectly identified as belonging to a category—for different threshold values. See figure 17.4 for an example.

The number that indicates how well the classifier performs is then the area under that curve. If that number is 0.5, it indicates that the classifier is performing no better than chance, and if that number is 1.0, it indicates perfect performance on the part of the classifier. Our preliminary analysis produced results in the 0.8 to 0.9 range, which indicates good classification. We hope to improve these numbers, but even at this level, it appears that the classifiers will be useful tools in categorizing publications along the translational research spectrum.

We plan to complete the analyses and are discussing pursuing funding to further extend this work. Several other CTSA programs have expressed interest in our work, and this will hopefully lead to either a broader collaboration on future directions or

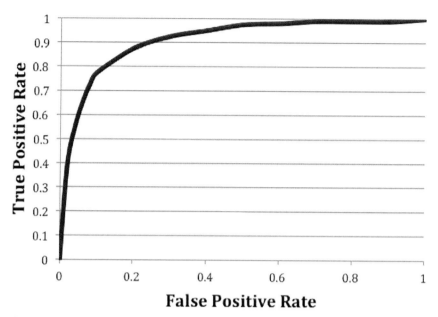

Figure 17.4. True positive rate plot versus false positive rate plot for different threshold values for a text classifier. The area under the curve is a measure of classifier performance.

a broad uptake of the definitions, checklist, and classifiers. By operationalizing the definitions of these categories of research along the translational spectrum, we hope that this work will provide a valuable tool for CTSA programs to evaluate the nature of their output and to demonstrate the impact of that output in moving research from the bench to the bedside and into the community.

FINAL THOUGHTS

While there was uptake within NYU's CTSI of the use of indirect and direct benefit as a way to track and report CTSI publications, this tracking was becoming increasingly unwieldy and was in all likelihood not sustainable as the numbers of publications continued to expand and my available time continued to contract. My initial idea of using machine learning to build classifiers to categorize publications along the translational research spectrum suffered from a naïveté around the nuts and bolts of machine learning as well as its limitations and the complexities of establishing definitions. For both of these projects, the key to success was collaboration.

For publication tracking, when I worked more closely with other CTSI personnel I was able to gain a better understanding of how others interacted with available data and what roles made sense for them to play in the tracking process. Different personnel were able to offer thoughts on where automation could be introduced, which allowed us to develop a viable and sustainable workflow.

In working with evaluators, informaticians, and other librarians on the publication classification project, I had to step outside of my silo, see other viewpoints, and sometimes find a way to translate between them. While this presented challenges, it was what allowed my initial bare idea to be fleshed out into a well-defined, feasible project. Those hurdles also helped me to have a greater understanding of the challenges of team science. And ultimately, having a collaboration that spanned skill sets and institutions increased the chances that the project could have a broad impact.

The projects described above are a sample of the work I've done with the NYU-HHC CTSI. Over the past five years, the range of my involvement in CTSI-related projects has grown considerably and includes:

- Spearheading the implementation of eagle-i research resource discovery system and profiles research-networking software at the institution;
- Coleading the development of a data catalog to describe widely used external data sets and data sets created by our researchers to facilitate data reuse and promote collaboration;
- Working with the CTSI participant recruitment working group on a novel idea for using the electronic health record (EHR) to facilitate connections between researchers and clinicians in order to enhance recruitment efforts;
- Contributing to the writing of the informatics section of our 2015 CTSA application; and
- Leading the writing of the team science section of the 2015 application and subsequently serving as program director for team science.

My involvement with the CTSI began with publication-related projects, a natural fit for a librarian. As I took on projects that had a broader information-management focus, the CTSI began to look to me to fill those types of needs. What I have seen in my experience with the NYU-HHC CTSI is that many needs emerge that do not seem to fall neatly under any person or program's strictly defined responsibilities. These gaps can cause the very research inefficiencies that the CTSA program seeks to remedy. With an expanded view of the librarian's role, the CTSI recognized that a librarian was best suited to address these needs when related to information management, flow, or discovery.

NOTES

1. Vieira D, McGowan R, McCrillis A, et al. The faculty bibliography project at the NYU School of Medicine. *Journal of Librarianship and Scholarly Communication*. 2014;2(3):eP1161.

2. Rubio DM. Common metrics to assess the efficiency of clinical research. *Eval Health Prof.* 2013 Dec;36(4):432–46.

3. Institute of Medicine. *The CTSA Program at NIH: Opportunities for Advancing Clinical and Translational Research.* Washington, DC: National Academies Press; 2013.

4. Pathfinder. Harvard Catalyst. https://catalyst.harvard.edu/pathfinder. Accessed July 23, 2015.

5. Translational Research, UT Southwestern, Dallas, TX. http://www.utsouthwestern.edu/research/translational-medicine/about/translational/index.html. Accessed July 23, 2015.

6. Khoury MJ, Gwinn M, Yoon PW, Dowling N, Moore CA, Bradley L. The continuum of translation research in genomic medicine: How can we accelerate the appropriate integration of human genome discoveries into health care and disease prevention? *Genet Med.* 2007 Oct;9(10):665–74.

7. Marmot M, Friel S, Bell R, Houweling TA, Taylor S. Closing the gap in a generation: Health equity through action on the social determinants of health. *Lancet* (London, England). 2008 Nov 8;372(9650):1661–69.

8. Waldman SA, Terzic A. Clinical and translational science: From bench-bedside to global village. *Clin Transl Sci.* 2010 Oct;3(5):254–57.

9. Blumberg RS, Dittel B, Hafler D, von Herrath M, Nestle FO. Unraveling the autoimmune translational research process layer by layer. *Nature Medicine.* 2012 Jan;18(1):35–41.

10. Gorter S, Rethans JJ, Schepbier A, et al. Developing case-specific checklists for standardized-patient-based assessments in internal medicine: A review of the literature. *Academic Medicine.* 2000 Nov;75(11):1130–37.

11. Vu NV, Marcy MM, Colliver JA, Verhulst SJ, Travis TA, Barrows HS. Standardized (simulated) patients accuracy in recording clinical-performance checklist items. *Medical Education.* 1992 Mar;26(2):99–104.

Index

About the Contributors

Roger A. Altizer Jr. is cofounder of Entertainment Arts and Engineering, the top ranked game design program in the nation, director of digital medicine for the Center for Medical Innovation, director of the GApp Lab (therapeutic games and applications), and former director of the Center for Interdisciplinary Art and Technology at the University of Utah. Roger earned his PhD in communications at Utah and specializes in game design education and participatory design. Creator of the Design Box, an inductive design methodology, Roger works to include audiences as designers in his work. A former games journalist, he is an internationally recognized speaker who has presented at industry conferences such as the Games Developer Conference and Penny Arcade eXpo and academic conferences such as the Digital Games Research Association and Foundations of Digital Games. He has made dozens of media appearances speaking on a variety of subjects ranging from games education and the social and legal issues of gaming.

Marci D. Brandenburg, MS, MSI, is the bioinformationist at the University of Michigan's Taubman Health Sciences Library. She works closely with the Department of Computational Medicine and Bioinformatics and the Bioinformatics Core in addition to supporting bioinformatics research on campus. She provides instruction on a variety of visualization tools, creates tool documentation, and coordinates a weekly tools and technology seminar. Before coming to the University of Michigan in 2010, she was the biosciences informationist at the National Cancer Institute–Frederick. Brandenburg holds an MS in biology from Ohio University and MSI from the University of Michigan and has worked for the National Wildlife Federation, the USDA Wildlife Services, and the University of Michigan's Medical School as a lab technician.

Celeste B. Choate has worked in public libraries for more than twenty-two years. She is the executive director of the Urbana Free Library in Urbana, Illinois, where she serves a community of 41,250 people. She was previously the associate director of services, collections, and access at the Ann Arbor District Library, where she was co-principal investigator on the National Institutes of Health grant Engaging the Community in Clinical Research. Choate received a master's in information and library studies from the University of Michigan.

Marisa L. Conte is the research and data informationist at the University of Michigan's (U-M) Taubman Health Sciences Library where she partners with researchers and administration to integrate library resources, services, and expertise into the research enterprise. She has worked with U-M's clinical and translational research community since 2007 and is a graduate of Wayne State University and proud alumna of the National Library of Medicine's Associate Fellowship Program. Her research interests include biomedical informatics, data management, team science, research ethics, and research policy.

Molly Dwyer-White has dedicated her career to community and patient engagement. She is manager of patient- and family-centered care for adult services at the University of Michigan Health System, where she works to build and support the infrastructure and tools for patients and families, health professionals, and hospital staff to work in active partnerships at various levels—point of care, organization design and policy, governance, and communication—to improve health, health care, and health equity. Dwyer-White formerly managed the development and steward-ship of the Michigan Institute for Clinical Research's Community Engagement Program and the Research Participant Recruitment Program, where she oversaw institutional approaches to building partnerships, improving clinical research recruitment, and effectively engaging communities and patients and practices in the translational research process via bidirectional dialogues.

Robert J. Engeszer, MLS, AHIP, is the associate director for translational research support at the Bernard Becker Medical Library at Washington University School of Medicine in St. Louis. His division develops programs and services targeted for each component of the translational research process including basic science support for labs and bench scientists; author services for scholarly communication and dissemination of research; health literacy and health communication services for community-engaged clinicians and researchers; and evaluation and assessment services to measure the impact of research and scholarly works.

Sally A. Gore, MS, MS LIS, is a research evaluation analyst for the University of Massachusetts Center for Clinical and Translational Science (CCTS) with responsibilities in development, implementation, and analysis of evaluation related to the programs and projects of the CCTS. Most immediately prior to this, she was an embedded research librarian and informationist at the Lamar Soutter Library, University of Massachusetts Medical School, serving on grant-funded clinical and community outreach research teams and providing information, data, and knowledge-management services for the projects. Gore earned her graduate degree in library and information science from Syracuse University and an MS in exercise physiology from Ithaca College (New York).

Karen E. Gutzman, MA, MSLS, is the impact and evaluation librarian for Galter Health Sciences Library at Northwestern University's Feinberg School of Medicine. Her responsibilities are to support individuals and groups in their understanding, assessment, visualization, and reporting of impactful outcomes of research and clinical care efforts. Gutzman works within the library's Metrics and Impact Core, which uses methods and services such as bibliometric analysis, social network analysis, alternative metrics, and micro–case studies to provide an understanding of research impact.

Kristi L. Holmes, PhD, is director of the Galter Health Sciences Library, director of evaluation for Northwestern University Clinical and Translational Sciences Institute, and associate professor of preventive medicine in the Division of Health and Biomedical Informatics at the Northwestern University Feinberg School of Medicine. Holmes focuses her research efforts on the development and application of information standards to enable interoperability and data exchange and leads a number of efforts related to metrics and research impact. She seeks to define new roles and opportunities for the modern biomedical research library in an increasingly informatics and data-driven environment.

Christina N. Kalinger graduated from the MEAE program at the University of Utah in May 2015. She currently lives in Boston and works as an associate producer for Harmonix, a video game studio specializing in musical and beat-matching games. She is also working independently on a project that investigates the potential usage of new VR technology for improving reflexes and reaction times in adults.

Leena N. Lalwani is an engineering librarian and the coordinator for engineering collections at the Art, Architecture, and Engineering Library (AAEL) at the University of Michigan. She is the liaison librarian for biomedical engineering, chemical engineering, materials science, naval architecture and marine engineering, and entrepreneurship. Lalwani is also the patent and trademarks expert for the library. She has been a librarian at University of Michigan since 1995 in various ranks. Prior to joining University of Michigan, she worked as librarian at Gelman Sciences and American Tobacco Company. Lalwani has an MLS degree from Catholic University of America and an MS in chemistry from the University of Mumbai.

266

Diana Nelson Louden is the biomedical and translational sciences librarian at the University of Washington Health Sciences Library in Seattle. In this position she works with the Institute of Translational Health Sciences where she is particularly involved in the KL2 Multidisciplinary Clinical Research Career Development Program. Louden also serves as a library liaison to several departments within the School of Medicine, providing instruction and research support to the faculty, students, and the staff. Prior to her academic appointment in 2012, she enjoyed a seventeen-year career as the biomedical and patent research librarian at ZymoGenetics, Inc., in Seattle.

Jennifer A. Lyon is the biomedical and translational research librarian at Stony Brook University Libraries. She has more than sixteen years of experience, previously working at the University of Florida and Vanderbilt University Medical Center. Her responsibilities have included supporting basic science, clinical, and translational researchers and course-integrated instruction and rounding with clinical units. Lyon holds an MS in molecular biology from the University of Wisconsin–Madison as well as her MLIS from the University of North Carolina–Greensboro. Her research interests include embedded librarianship, librarian professional development in clinical medicine, bioinformatics, systematic reviews, and health literacy.

Dorene S. Markel is the director of the Brehm Center at the University of Michigan Health System (U-MHS), which is focused on transforming the way research and collaborations are undertaken utilizing diabetes as a platform. She is the coordinator of the Brehm Coalition, a "dream team" of ten senior scientists in type 1 diabetes research from nine universities. Markel holds a faculty appointment in the medical school's Department of Learning Health Sciences and is playing a key role in initiating a learning health system approach to diabetes care at U-MHS. Markel received a master's in human genetics, specializing in genetic counseling, from the University of Michigan Medical School and a master's in health services administration from the University of Michigan School of Public Health.

Emily S. Mazure, MSI, AHIP, has been the biomedical research liaison librarian at Duke University Medical Center Library and Archives since November 2010. Before she joined Duke, she was an education and research librarian at Tompkins-McCaw Health Science Library at Virginia Commonwealth University; previously she was a libraries fellow at North Carolina State University. In her current position, Mazure provides targeted support and services to biomedical researchers in the Duke community. She has supported Duke University's National Institutes of Health public access compliance since 2012 through the development of educational resources and compliance monitoring.

Brenda L. Minor is the relationship manager for REDCap (Research Electronic Data Capture), a program of the Vanderbilt Institute for Clinical and Translational

Research. Minor has worked with REDCap in various capacities since 2008 and is currently leader member of the REDCap support team, liaison to the REDCap consortium, and key support for Vanderbilt end users and their collaborators. Prior to working in research, she held management positions in the import, entertainment, and service industries. Brenda holds a BS in liberal studies (with an emphasis in communications and corporate management) from Middle Tennessee State University. She enjoys being involved in all things REDCap, including administration of the REDCap Shared Library and other collaborative work including an Ebola monitoring project and new Precision Medicine initiatives.

Valrie I. Minson is chair of University of Florida's Marston Science Library, responsible for all aspects of service development, collaborative development and partnerships, and research and information reporting supports. From 2009 to 2011, she served as national and local implementation lead for the VIVO: National Networking of Scientists–funded grant and, from 2005 to 2014, served as an agricultural sciences librarian. Her research focuses on the changing role of librarians and the potential for stronger collaborations, whether through supporting faculty research reporting, developing and implementing new discovery tools, or coordinating scientific art contests. She has a bachelor's from University of South Florida and a master's in library science from Florida State University.

Fatima M. Mncube-Barnes is the executive director of the Health Sciences Library at Howard University. She supported the Clinical and Translational Science Award (CTSA) program as a bioinformatician and later managed the Meharry Medical College Library. Mncube-Barnes earned an EdD from the University of Tennessee, an AB in organization behavior and management from Brown University, an EdM in technology, innovation, and education from Harvard, an MPH in public health informatics from the University of Illinois in Chicago, and an MSIS from the University of Tennessee in Knoxville. Her research interests include technology integration in medical education, public health informatics, dental informatics, clinical research, and professional development.

Hannah F. Norton is reference and liaison librarian at the University of Florida Health Science Center Library, serving primarily as liaison to the College of Veterinary Medicine, the Department of Medicine, and the College of Medicine Class of 2019. She holds a BA in biology from Carleton College and an MS in information studies from the University of Texas at Austin. Norton's research interests include library support for e-science and data curation, library as place, and evaluation of various academic library services.

William Olmstadt is the associate director of the health sciences library and a tenured associate librarian in the Department of Medical Library Science at Louisiana State University Health Sciences Center Shreveport in Shreveport, Louisiana. He has worked in libraries since 1994. He earned an MSLS from the University of Kentucky and a graduate degree in public health from the University of Texas Health Science Center at Houston. He is a distinguished member of the Academy of Health Information Professionals (AHIP) of the Medical Library Association. He has written and presented on the broad topics of instruction and consumer health in health science libraries.

Lisa A. Palmer, MSLS, AHIP, is the institutional repository librarian for the Lamar Soutter Library at the University of Massachusetts Medical School. She oversees eScholarship@UMMS, the medical school's repository and publishing system for digital research and scholarship. In this role she serves as an editor for the *Journal of eScience Librarianship* and other publications. She also provides support for scholarly communication activities, open access, author rights, copyright, research data management, and National Institutes of Health public access compliance. She earned her graduate degree in library science from Simmons College in Boston. Prior to joining the University of Massachusetts, Palmer was a corporate librarian for Digital Equipment Corporation, Compaq Computer Corporation, and Hewlett-Packard.

Cathy C. Sarli, MLS, AHIP, is the senior librarian of evaluation services for the Translational Research Support Division at Becker Medical Library, Washington University School of Medicine in St. Louis. She specializes in research and publishing issues, assessment of research impact, and compliance with public access mandates. Sarli serves as the project lead for the Becker Model for Assessment of Research Impact and is also a member of the Tracking and Evaluation Team for the Washington University Institute of Clinical and Translational Sciences (ICTS).

Kate Saylor is an informationist at the Taubman Health Sciences Library (THL) at the University of Michigan. She currently works with the School of Nursing, School of Public Health's Health Behavior and Health Education Department, and the Office of Public Health Practice. In addition to these schools and centers, she also supports the academic and clinical needs within the University of Michigan Health System's departments of pediatrics and ophthalmology and visual sciences. Saylor previously worked in outreach for THL promoting the health of the community by way of improving access to high-quality health information, with an emphasis on underserved communities and the elimination of health disparities.

Pamela L. Shaw is biosciences and bioinformatics librarian at the Galter Health Sciences Library of the Feinberg School of Medicine of Northwestern University. She holds a bachelor's in psychobiology and master's degrees in library and information science and computational biology and bioinformatics. She was employed for twenty years as a neuroanatomy and neuropathology technician before moving to Galter

Library in January of 2006. Shaw has coauthored papers in neuroscience, genomics, and computational biology. She provides instruction and consultation in bibliographic management, National Institutes of Health public access policy compliance, and bioinformatics at Galter Library.

Jean P. Shipman is director of the Spencer S. Eccles Health Sciences Library, the MidContinental Region and National Training Office of the National Network of Libraries of Medicine, and director for information transfer at the Center for Medical Innovation at the University of Utah. She is also adjunct professor in the Department of Biomedical Informatics, School of Medicine, at the University of Utah. She served as president of the Medical Library Association for 2006–2007 and promoted health literacy as her primary presidential initiative, including creating a national health literacy curriculum. Her professional interests are health literacy, scholarly communications, library administration, innovation, and lean libraries.

Judith E. Smith is an informationist at the Taubman Health Sciences Library at the University of Michigan, Ann Arbor. Her primary roles include integrating information services and resources into the North Campus Research Complex (NCRC), which focuses on interdisciplinary and translational research, and into the Department of Health Policy and Management in the School of Public Health. Previously, Smith served as the virtual library services coordinator within the Entrepreneurial Library Program (ELP) of the Sheridan Libraries at the Johns Hopkins University and worked in the philanthropic sector as a research associate at the Carnegie Corporation of New York.

Amy M. Suiter, MS, MLS, is a scholarly publishing librarian at the Bernard Becker Medical Library at Washington University School of Medicine in St. Louis. She is a member of the tracking and evaluation team for the Washington University Institute of Clinical and Translational Sciences (ICTS). Suiter serves as comanager of the library's institutional repository and provides support in the areas of copyright, public access mandates, and evaluation of scholarly productivity and impact. She generates h-index reports, social network analysis maps, and publication reports for scholars and departments on campus.

Alisa Surkis is the translational science librarian for the Health Sciences Library at New York University's (NYU) School of Medicine. She serves as the director of team science and a member of the evaluation working group for the NYU-HHC Clinical and Translational Science Institute and as a member of the library's data services team. Through these roles she has supported and developed a number of systems and programs to promote collaboration, including research networking systems and an institutional data catalog, and has worked both within her institution and with other Clinical and Translational Science Award (CTSA) hubs to develop innovative evaluation methodologies.

Michele R. Tennant, PhD, MLIS, is associate director for the Health Science Center Library, University of Florida (UF), and has provided reference, liaison, and instructional services to UF faculty and students since 1995, with a focus on outreach, teaching, and library-based bioinformatics support. Tennant was the University of Florida lead for local outreach on the VIVO project and presented at numerous library and scientific conferences on this research tool. She is currently funded to lead a team of library faculty to provide HIV/AIDS information outreach to clinicians, the general public, social service organizations, educators, and other librarians.

Patricia L. Thibodeau, MLS, MBA, AHIP, FMLA, is associate dean of library services and archives and for the Medical Center Library and Archives, Duke University. Prior to Duke, Thibodeau was director of information and media services at the Mountain Area Health Education Center in Asheville, North Carolina; earlier, the library director and research administrator at the Women and Infants Hospital of Rhode Island in Providence. She has been involved in the National Institutes of Health public access policy development, implementation, and compliance efforts for Duke since 2005, working with Duke University's Clinical and Translational Science Award (CTSA) faculty and staff since 2007 and developing strategies for tracking faculty and research publications for more than ten years.

Mychal A. Voorhees, MA, is the health literacy and community outreach coordinator at the Bernard Becker Medical Library at Washington University School of Medicine in St. Louis. She coordinates the library's Communicating for Health program, which provides health literacy and health communication services across campus. Voorhees's professional interests include improving health communication education for providers and simplifying complex information for lay audiences. In addition to her work at the library, she also teaches professional communication courses for pharmacy students.

Elizabeth C. Whipple is a research librarian at the Ruth Lilly Medical Library of Indiana University School of Medicine (IUSM) in Indianapolis. Her work on information discovery includes bibliometric analysis through supporting and analyzing the publication output of the Indiana Clinical and Translational Sciences Institute (CTSI), as well as the patterns of coauthorship across Indiana CTSI member institutions. She also works with several IUSM departments to enhance their education and support their research through the development and creation of discipline-specific information portals, knowledge-management consultation, and end-user social media tools.